T0209882

Praise for *Writing Yoga*

"A warm, compassionate, and intimate guide to the journey through words and yoga postures to the vastness that lies beyond them. Through his own personal explorations of yoga and journal-writing, Bruce Black illuminates the path of self-discovery, creativity, and transformation."
—Anne Cushman, author of *Enlightenment for Idiots: A Novel*

"For anyone who's looking for answers, Bruce Black's *Writing Yoga* will absolutely help you find them—on the page, and on the mat."
—August Gold, author of *Prayer Partners*

"I have been writing and studying yoga for years now but never thought to join these two passions until I read Bruce Black's account of his own journey. He says yoga can be a catalyst for change. So can reading this honest, profound, and compassionate book!"
—Louise Hawes, author of *Anteaters Don't Dream*, Faculty, MFA in Writing for Children and Young Adults, Vermont College of Fine Arts

"The practice of yoga is a process of uncovering our thoughts, beliefs, and assumed limitations, be they physical, emotional,

or mental. In this warm, personal book, Bruce Black reveals how his own journey in yoga and writing has brought clarity and direction to his life. Try his suggestions; I have. And see if you don't feel more at ease and present with your life."
—Judith Hanson Lasater, Ph.D., P.T., yoga teacher and coauthor of *What We Say Matters*

WRITING YOGA

WRITING YOGA

A Guide to Keeping a Practice Journal

Bruce Black

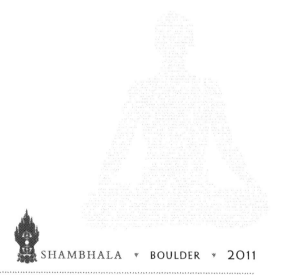

SHAMBHALA ▼ BOULDER ▼ 2011

Shambhala Publications, Inc.
2129 13th Street
Boulder, Colorado 80302
www.shambhala.com

Editors: Holly Hammond, Linda Cogozzo
Design: Gopa & Ted2, Inc.
Author Photo: Courtesy of Bruce Black
Text set in Weiss

Printed in the United States of America

♾ This edition is printed on acid-free paper that meets the American National Standards Institute Z39.48 Standard.
♻ Shambhala Publications makes every effort to print on recycled paper. For more information please visit www.shambhala.com
Shambhala Publications is distributed worldwide by Penguin Random House, Inc., and its subsidiaries.

The Library of Congress catalogues the original edition of this book as follows:
Black, Bruce. Writing yoga: a guide to keeping a practice journal / Bruce Black. 1st ed.
Berkley, CA: Rodmell Press, 2011.
xiii, 159 p. ; 23 cm.
B132.Y6 B613 2011
ISBN 9781930485280 (pbk.)

In memory of my father, David B. Black.
May his memory be a blessing.

Contents

Acknowledgments

The first four letters of the word "journal" are the same as the first four letters of the word "journey." They spell *jour,* the French word for "day" or "daily." The process of keeping a journal, as I have over the past few years, is one of making a journey, an interior journey, which unfolds every day from the moment you open your notebook and begin writing.

During the years that I spent writing this book, I was assisted in my journey by many people who were kind enough to extend a helping hand. Their enthusiasm for this project and their faith in my ability to complete it were great gifts. I feel surrounded by their love and support.

I owe a special debt of gratitude to the following people:

My yoga teachers, Jaye Martin and Rita Knorr, who have become more than teachers, and who knew before I did that practicing yoga and keeping a journal would help me expand in ways that I could not have imagined. Their devotion to yoga, and their belief in the endless possibilities of life, continue to serve as inspiration for my writing and my yoga practice.

Vesna Petrovich, Corey Terzo, and Nancy Zampella—all dedicated teachers who I studied with at Garden of the Heart Yoga Center and who helped me find my way.

The students in Rita's class, who gathered on Tuesday mornings and who shared their lives so generously each week, especially Lena and Pat, who offered more support (and humor) than they knew, and who continue offering their support as we prepare for our weekly classes with Jaye.

Paula Morris, a student in Rita's class who now teaches at GOH, and Jeanne Panka, a fellow student in Jaye's class, who read portions of this manuscript in its earliest stage, when many of the ideas were mere shadows, and offered the same loving encouragement and support that they offer in class whenever I find myself in a difficult pose.

Randall Buskirk, for his willingness to share insights into yoga and writing over lunch at Mo's place on the Trail, and for teaching in his class at GOH, where I'm a frequent drop-in on Friday mornings, about the importance of patience and listening to your heart.

Betsey Downing, Ph.D., the founder of Garden of the Heart Yoga Center, whose vision of life and its myriad possibilities guides each class, and John Friend, the founder of Anusara Yoga, who I've never met but whose spirit pervades the classes at GOH.

My teachers and friends in the MFA in Writing Program at Vermont College, as well as other writers, who have so generously shared their knowledge of the craft and their insights into the writing process over the years: Graham Salisbury, Jacqueline Woodson, Norma Fox Mazer, Marion Dane Bauer, Louise

Hawes, Phyllis Root, Ellen Howard, Chris Lynch, Sharon Bryant, Cynthia Bassett, Anita Riggio, Judy Kuns, Carmela A. Martino, Carolyn Crimi, Dave Masterton, Chuck Entwistle, Jack O'Rourke, Steven Schnur, David Shifren, Amy Lang, and B.J. Chute.

Donald Moyer and Linda Cogozzo, the talented copublishers of Rodmell Press.

Rick Black, my brother, for always looking at life's challenges—especially when it comes to finding the time to write—with humor and patience, for never failing to break into a hearty laugh of disbelief whenever I describe myself attempting a difficult, pretzel-like yoga pose, and for his unwavering faith that, even when it appears that I may have taken a wrong turn, I'll find my way again.

Susan, my loving (and lovely) and ever-patient wife, and Madeline, our wise-beyond-her-years daughter, for their unflagging enthusiasm for this project and for their daily support (and suggestions over dinner) during the many months that it took to complete the manuscript, for doing the extra loads of laundry and dishes that I was supposed to do, and for running to the grocery store for another loaf of bread or gallon of milk while I was hunched over my desk, lost in a maze of revisions.

David B. Black, my dear father, who would have loved to see the publication of this book but who died on June 7, 2009, at the age of ninety-four, six months before I submitted the completed draft for publication. His spirit guides my work even now, these many months after his death.

And a special note of gratitude to you, dear reader, for joining me on this journey.

Introduction: Getting Started

Give yourself permission to make mistakes, to be.
—FROM MY JOURNAL

....

A journal is another prop—like a block, a belt, a blanket—for you
to use in your yoga practice. It can help you open to another side
of yourself. By keeping a journal in conjunction with your yoga
practice, you'll develop a greater sense of mindfulness and pur-
pose, and through your newfound focus you'll uncover insights
about yourself and your practice that may surprise you.

This book is a tool to help you get started with your practice
journal. In each chapter I share some of my explorations on the
mat and reflect on how my yoga practice, combined with keeping a journal, led to insights into my life. Each chapter's themes
can be woven into the rhythms of your own yoga and journal
practice, so you can dip into the book chapter by chapter or
read it through in its entirety before going back to explore the
themes that resonate more strongly for you.

....

You'll find exercises at the end of each chapter to help you further explore the chapter's topics as they relate to your life. Feel free to follow the exercises or design your own set of questions after finishing a chapter. Through the process of writing on a regular basis, you will discover what works and what doesn't, so you can develop your own journal practice.

First Steps

In high school in the late 1960s, whenever I gazed down at a blank sheet of paper in the hope of writing a story or poem, I felt my insides wither and my mind go numb. I was frozen with fear that my teachers might consider whatever I wrote foolish and inane.

Fear of writing was such a huge obstacle early on—fear of embarrassing myself in front of my classmates, fear of ridicule by teachers, fear of not having anything to say, fear that my voice might reveal my uncertainty about the story that I was trying to tell—that often I turned away from the page before writing anything at all. In those years, many sheets of paper were crumpled into the wastebasket or tossed onto the floor. The journals I started would be abandoned after I wrote a page or two. Those early years of writing were attempts, I realize now, to learn how to use language and to find my voice, a voice that felt natural and unpretentious. I could hear the voice inside my head but could not reproduce it on paper.

It was in college in the early 1970s that I first realized the power of keeping a journal. One of my English literature professors assigned us the task of keeping a journal about the books we read in class, a diary, really, of our thoughts as we read through the assignments that semester. In that journal I discovered a different kind of writing, a *private* voice rather than a public voice, and an ease in finding words and putting them down on paper that I'd never experienced before. My favorite time for writing in the journal was at night after my roommate went to sleep and the dorm was quiet. I'd sit at my desk with the lamp on low and listen to my inner voice in a way that was impossible when I wrote end-of-semester papers for other classes. Writing in my journal, I was no longer worried about how someone else—a teacher, another classmate—might judge my words. Writing became a way to discover what I was thinking and feeling, and how my thoughts and feelings related to the books our class was reading, and ultimately to the world beyond books.

That was the first time, really, that I heard my voice. The voice in my journal was so personal, so intimate and honest, that it scared me. It made me feel vulnerable, open to the world. And after graduating from college in 1976, I put aside journal writing. I was too busy figuring out how to make a living with words, imagining how I might craft stories that would appear in the pages of *The New Yorker* beside the work of my favorite authors—Cheever, Updike, Nabokov, and Singer.

Without realizing that I had "found" my voice in my journal, I went in search of it elsewhere. Instead of looking within, I looked at how other writers crafted their stories. I thought I might find my voice in the daily work of writing for a local newspaper. But I found that newspaper writing, like writing term papers, demanded a public rather than a private voice, a voice more formal than intimate, and I struggled with journalism because the writing felt false, full of facts but lacking the emotional undercurrents that pulled me into fiction.

I forgot the private voice that I'd found in my journal until my mother died in 1977. During her illness, I began keeping journals again—raw, intimate diaries about my feelings toward death and cancer and God, why suffering exists in the world and how to hold on to faith in the face of unrelenting pain. Those journals were written late at night or early in the morning before anyone else in the house was awake. They were the beginning of my attempt to reconnect with the voice that I'd first heard in college.

In the years after my mother's death, I switched jobs from newspaper reporter to stock clerk in a bookstore, then entered publishing to become an editor. I began placing stories in magazines and newspapers. Throughout those years I kept pocket-sized journals with me and during lunch spent hours writing, filling pages with questions about how to write and what to write, gaining a sense of myself again and what was important to me, what I felt passionate about. Those journals were the precursors to the journal that I began keeping in 2007 to explore my yoga practice.

Until 2007 I had kept journals off and on, losing interest, picking up a thread again, using a journal to keep track of well-written or moving passages in books or to record something of interest that I saw that day, experimenting with story ideas or ways of presenting a story. Eventually those journals served as draft notebooks in which I worked out plot or character issues. The entries were less about my own thoughts and feelings, more about the thoughts and feelings of my characters.

But when we moved to a new home in Florida, I began taking yoga classes at Garden of the Heart Yoga Center, where the teachers practice a form of yoga known as Anusara. By 2007 I'd found my way into Rita's class and was touched when she handed a blank journal to each student and encouraged us to use them to deepen our practice and understanding of yoga. So I began keeping a journal again, one that focused on my yoga practice, on what I learned from the poses and challenges on the mat, as well as on how yoga seemed to change the way that I understood myself, my relationships to other people and to the world.

Each time I stepped onto my mat as part of my home practice, I opened my journal for a few minutes and jotted down my thoughts instead of immediately beginning the poses. Writing in the journal became a way for me to notice more closely what was happening in my life—what was going smoothly, what seemed hard—and how I was responding or failing to respond to the challenges. Little by little, the pages of the journal filled with thoughts and feelings, and I began sharing some of the pages with Rita. One day she asked if I'd share some thoughts with the class. Then Rita suggested that we collaborate on teaching a class together to encourage more people to develop their own journal practice. As a way of further exploring the relationship between journal writing and yoga, I started my own blog, and blogging helped me find the voice that I needed to write this book.

The journal and the mat are places where I can think through problems that I'm facing without judging myself and without feeling pressure to solve the problems. I can just let the problem out and consider it, the way I might look at a tree or rock, without trying to "solve" it. And in the process of looking, I'll see something that I hadn't noticed before, the hint of a path, the suggestion of an answer.

Taking Your First Steps

Just as the practice of yoga encourages you to hear and trust your inner voice, so too does the practice of keeping a journal. Writing every day can help you work past the distracting noises of the world so you can listen more closely to the voice that can be found deep inside you. Day after day, as your thoughts appear beneath your pen as it moves across the page, you'll begin to hear your voice emerge out of the silence. That voice will teach you what you need to know in your yoga practice and in your life.

The first step to hearing your voice is learning to listen to the sounds around you. Writing about what you hear in the world—the very noises that distract you or irritate you or make you angry or frustrated—is the first step to recognizing the difference between those noises and your voice. In the process of noticing and writing down your observations and thoughts, you'll move from noticing the voices of doubt, resistance, and fear that may distract you from hearing your own voice to noticing the voice that pulls you deeper inside. Your voice is a refuge from the noise of the world, and your journal can become a sanctuary, a special place where you can hear the music of your soul through the daily act of writing and reflecting in your journal.

This type of journal writing takes skill, practice, and patience, just as yoga practice requires skill and understanding as you make your way into different poses. For some writers, the blank page can be an intimidating obstacle to putting down those first words. But like the shimmering surface of a lake or pond, once you break the surface, you can play and enjoy your time in the water. How can you break the surface of the blank page? You might consider playing with lines or dots or doodles, simply taking pleasure in the flow of ink and the movement of your hand across the page. Eventually words will appear as you become more comfortable with the page in front of you. As you approach each exercise, if you don't know what to write, follow the advice that Natalie Goldberg offers in her book, *Writing Down the Bones*, and write: "I don't know what to write." Keep writing the phrase until another phrase or word comes into your mind, and then write that word or phrase. Notice if you feel blocked or closed, and describe your feelings on the page.

After you've written for at least five minutes, close your journal, put down your pen, and shut your eyes. Notice if you feel more open to the world, to yourself. Whatever you notice, you can reflect on how you came to feel that way in your next journal entry. In time, you'll want to write for as long as you feel inspired to. But in the beginning, try to write for at least five minutes each day, either before or after your asana practice.

Being Yourself

Your voice has many layers, many disguises. How do you know which is your true voice? The process of finding it involves a challenging search and demands that you ask yourself questions that reveal who you really are. For instance, is your true voice the whining, complaining voice that you hear when you don't get what you want or when life doesn't go the way you think it should? Or is it the voice of authority that you use in your job or with your children? Or the voice of submission that you use with a parent or spouse, teacher or supervisor? Perhaps it's the voice of joy you hear when playing in the pool or balancing in Tree Pose for the first time, or the voice of despair when you've lost something—or someone—dear to your heart.

You may find that your voice contains all of these voices. Your journal will give you an opportunity to hear each voice and explore it in new ways. If you're like me, you'll find that exploring each voice leads to the discovery that beneath each voice is another voice, a voice that notices how you assume the role of all the other voices and how each voice reflects a different aspect of your personality at different times in your life. What is crucial is that you notice how these other voices emerge or evolve out of that deeper, unique voice, so you can pay more attention to that deeper voice guiding all the others. That's the voice that forms the core of your being.

Keeping a journal, like practicing yoga, lets you be yourself without needing to assume a role or a disguise. You can be yourself on the page; you can hear what you're really thinking and feeling. The emotions that arise as you write, the sensations that your body transmits, are raw, unfiltered, uncensored. There's no need to pretend you're feeling one thing to please anyone, no need to say words that you don't mean for fear of offending or hurting someone's feelings. Your journal, like your mat, is your refuge, a place where you can let down your guard and discover who you really are and celebrate that discovery. It will help you explore the question: Who am I?

FROM MY JOURNAL

 Is the practice of yoga merely a series of poses to stretch and strengthen one's muscles? Or is there a spiritual element that makes the poses more than simple exercise? This question remains at the root of my practice: is yoga exercise or spiritual quest? The answer, perhaps, can be found somewhere between the two extremes. Yoga brings together—or links—the spirit and the physical in new and unusual ways. It's a challenge, though, to find spiritual insight in a pose, to draw a lesson from pushing oneself into new or unfamiliar territory. The feeling is much like setting off in a new direction, not knowing exactly where you'll end up. And the point of the poses, I suspect, is to help us "see" the connection to our spiritual energy and the larger energy of the universe, so we can learn to trust that force, even when it's difficult to discern, even when we don't know how it can possibly lead us to where we're meant to be.

What You'll Need

You'll need something to write on and a pen (although some people prefer to keep their journals on a computer). You can buy the most expensive leather-bound journal or the cheapest cardboard-covered notebook. You can use lined or unlined, white or yellow paper. You can use a spiral notebook or loose-leaf folder or legal pad or drawing paper. You can use a journal small enough to fit in your back pocket or one the size of a laptop computer. Which do you feel most comfortable writing in?

I prefer the least expensive notebooks, usually made out of recycled paper and cardboard. I shy away from the more expensive, overly elaborate journals, the ones with thick, leather-tooled covers and gilt-edged paper. They're just too beautiful, and their beauty makes me think that the words that fill their pages need to be as beautiful and perfect as the journals. So I look for the cheapest notebooks I can find. The low cost lets me feel that I can write whatever I want and make mistakes and take detours and backtrack and follow wrong turns without worrying about the outcome.

The practice of journaling is all about process—the process of putting words on paper, the process of thinking and sifting through layers of memories and experiences to make discoveries and gain insights. It's not about what you produce. Like many writers, I rarely reread what I write in my journals. That's because it's in the process of writing—the actual physical act of writing—that you'll make discoveries. That's the point of keeping a journal—not the product, but the process. (Of course, it's fine if you decide to reread what you've written later on.)

What will help you get the words on paper? Start with one kind of pen or pencil, and, if that doesn't work, experiment with another. Take risks, use your imagination, play with different kinds of instruments, and find the one that feels the best in your hand. If you enjoy doodling before writing, go ahead and doodle. If you want to draw stick figures or cartoons or jot notes in the margins of your journal (or in this book), why shouldn't you? Cross-hatchings? Tic-tac-toe? Why not? You might even want to use your journal as a collage and paste inspiring quotes or funny pictures on the pages to help you get started the next time you open it to write. Or, for that matter, use the pages of your journal to express gratitude for the people and blessings in your life, with photos or mementos to help prompt your thoughts.

Do you prefer words that appear in bold, forceful lines? Then use a thicker, bolder pen. If you like the moodiness of gray, switch to a pencil or even a thin piece of charcoal. Or maybe you're feeling raw emotionally, and only a red pen will satisfy you this morning. Which color would best reflect your emotional state as you write? Pick one. Explore the way each pen brings out different emotions and thoughts, and enjoy the process of experimenting.

In my journals, I use pens with different colored inks—pink, turquoise, purple, green—depending on the way I feel on a given day. I love the way the colorful entries look next to each other after a week or a month. They remind me of a patchwork quilt or a collection of building blocks, and they give me a sense of making something, each passage contributing its unique design to the emerging story. But there are also times when I need to see multiple pages of black words, or blue. And on occasion I like to write in pencil, because I need to know that I can erase the words, even if I never do.

Are you a morning person or a late-night owl? Do you like tea or coffee? Do you prefer solitude or crowds? These kinds of questions and your answers will help you decide where and when you might like to journal: alone on your mat in a bedroom or sitting in a comfortable chair at a bookstore café. The process of deciding when and where to journal—thinking about it, but better yet, writing about your preferences—is part of the process of learning to listen to your inner voice. You may not need a lot of time—five, ten minutes to start—but you do need time, preferably when you won't be distracted or interrupted by children or ringing phones that must be answered. You may find it convenient to journal about yoga during lunch breaks rather than after finishing a yoga session. Or you may not want to leave your mat before completing an entry about that session and the thoughts and feelings that the poses evoked in you.

After you've kept a journal for a while, you may find that you're exploring multiple ideas and feel compelled to write not just about yoga but about work or raising children or relating to parents or interacting with your partner. Some writers find that keeping more than one journal at a time helps them focus on a particular issue or theme more clearly than keeping a single journal. Create your own journal practice so that it serves you.

Writing Without Rules

What should you write in your journal? It's different for everyone. Some people before starting to write like to settle on a theme or ask a question, such as why they might lack confidence to kick upside down into Headstand, or why they become angry in certain situations or with certain people. And then they use the journal to explore those questions or themes.

Other people write free-form journals, collections of random thoughts that come up in the process of writing. Just as each pose can lead to unexpected insights on the way to the next pose, so too can your words if you let them flow just to see what comes. They can help you learn what you're really thinking beneath the surface of consciousness.

Remember: There are no rules. You are free to write about whatever interests you or puzzles you or makes you wonder or gives you joy. Your journal is like your personal treasure box, a special place where you can put whatever you want: thoughts, emotions, sensations, observations, ideas, stories, memories, fears, hopes, dreams. You can explore whatever you want in whatever way you want without apology or explanation or plan.

FROM MY JOURNAL

Sometimes yoga—the idea of yoga—seems too demanding. My mind isn't prepared to explore the sensations that my muscles will experience. Or else I'm too tired to sustain a pose for long, never mind set my intention or declare a theme. Most of the time, I don't have a theme. And I don't know how to find one. I see only a blank slate. But I know that at the end of the yoga session, I will

feel relaxed thanks to the deep breathing, the muscle stretches.
And there's something more, too: a connection with something
larger than myself, a force bigger than my own spirit.

JOURNAL PRACTICE: GETTING STARTED

Are you ready to get started? Here are two exercises to help you
begin writing. You can come back to them, time and again, to
approach them from a different angle, a new perspective.

> ► Once you've selected a journal and pen and decided on a
> place to write, and you're sitting in a comfortable position,
> take a moment to look more closely at your journal. What
> drew you to this particular one? Take the time now to note
> its size, the color of the cover, and any designs or illustra-
> tions that make it unique. Run your hand over the spine,
> then open the journal and touch the blank pages. Lift the
> pages to your nose and smell the paper. As you inhale, can
> you smell the tree that the paper was made from and the
> woods where the tree once grew? Can you feel as if you
> are that tree and feel the rain falling on your leaves and
> the sunlight warming your branches? Listen to the sound
> of the leaves rustling in the wind, the tree limbs bending
> and creaking. As you turn the blank pages and feel the soft
> paper beneath your fingertips, imagine the paper as leaves
> that you've picked off the forest floor and pressed into the
> pages of the book you're holding.

Listening and imagining in this way expands your understanding of yourself in relationship to the world around you. Everything that you see or feel or taste or smell—the rain lashing your windshield as you drive to work, the drop of hot coffee that you spilled from your mug as you lifted it off your desk, the peach that you cut into sections for your cereal at breakfast—can serve as a subject to write about. By listening (and I mean listening with all your senses) you can feel deeply what it means to be physically present and connected to the world.

Now listen to the sounds around you. If you're in your bedroom or kitchen, take a moment to hear the noises inside and outside the room. If you're in a coffee shop, listen to what's happening in the space around you. If you hear a voice that suggests that this exercise is foolish and a waste of time, note that voice and what it's saying. If you hear a voice suggesting that you hear nothing and have nothing to write, note that voice. If you spend a few minutes—say, five at the most—you'll begin to distinguish the sounds around you. Voices, car horns, ambulances, garbage trucks, piped-in music, the hiss of an air conditioner, the thrum of a furnace, a child's cry, the sound of the wind, the drumming of raindrops on a windowpane. Just listen.

When you've spent a few minutes listening, open your journal and begin describing the noises you heard. Write about what you smelled or tasted or felt, too. Simply make a list of things, if you feel that's as much as you can write down at this time. Or let your imagination take you further, and explore how the noises made you feel and which noises helped you move into a contemplative state so you could begin writing and which noises seemed distracting and prevented you from putting words down on paper.

When you're finished writing, close your journal without rereading what you've written, put down your pen, and just listen again. What do you notice? And how did writing about the noises change or deepen your understanding of the noises around you and your relationship to them? If you would like to continue the exercise, you can spend some time responding to these questions (or asking your own questions). Or simply end the session with the knowledge that you've started your journal, and leave these questions as prompts to begin your next session.

▶ As you spend more and more time listening to the sounds around you, you'll begin to distinguish external noises from the internal voices that you hear throughout your day, which you may no longer notice because they've become so familiar. Just as you spent time noticing the noises around you, you can begin noticing the voices you hear inside your head, the voices that provide a kind of running commentary to whatever you're doing, and start differentiating one from another. Identify those voices that are negative and critical of what you do and those voices that are positive and supportive of your actions.

Again, it's important just to listen and not judge what you hear. Let the voice have its say. If it's a negative or severely critical voice, it may prove difficult to remain open enough so that you can actually hear it instead of dismissing it. And if it's a positive voice, an overly enthusiastic supporter of your actions, it may be hard to remain neutral in its presence. But that's the aim of this listening exercise. You simply want to welcome each voice. Let it speak, and listen respectfully to what it has to say, without judging it or concluding that you'd prefer not to hear it. Just listen. What do you hear?

Once you've identified these voices, the voices that you may have heard your entire life but hadn't really listened to until this moment, open your journal and begin describing them. What do the voices sound like? How often do you hear them? When do these particular voices seem most willing to speak? Do the voices remind you of people you know or have known? And how do the various voices make you feel? This last is perhaps the most important question to ask, because it will lead you to a deeper understanding of the difference between those voices and your true voice, the voice that's already beginning to emerge on the pages of your journal.

1: Opening Up

Some days you may find a flood of ideas and words;
other days only a trickle.
—FROM MY JOURNAL

....

I came to yoga—or yoga came to me—in the roundabout way that happens for many men my age. Five years ago, I was turning fifty and slowly coming to realize that my middle-aged bones and muscles weren't designed to run over pavement for five or ten miles a day. They required gentler, less stressful forms of exercise than they had withstood for years.

From my early years in high school, through college, and for more than fifteen years afterward—for more than twenty years—I had devoted myself to running, three to five miles a day, more on weekends. It wasn't just how I stayed in shape. It was how I stayed in touch with myself, my inner thoughts, my body. But now my legs, especially my knees, were beginning to show signs of wear.

By the time we'd moved south to Sarasota from Philadelphia

....

so my wife could take a position on the faculty of a local college, I could no longer run without pain. So, instead of running, I started bicycling and swimming. Each was low-impact, meaning that to exercise I didn't have to strain my knees or other joints. The ease of pedaling, the buoyancy of the water, kept my knees from aching. But neither form of exercise really served as an adequate substitute for running. Without the ability to run, I felt as if something were missing from my life.

For so many years I had relied on running as a way to quiet my mind. If I was angry or disturbed, I could leave my troubles behind by pulling on my running shoes and heading out in all sorts of weather—rain, sleet, snow—to go a few miles. I loved the time alone at dawn or dusk, the chance to sort through questions and doubts and hear myself think, to follow my thoughts wherever they might lead.

Bicycling, in contrast to running, requires a certain awareness of where you're riding on the road, especially as cars speed past only inches away from the bike lane. You can never really lose yourself in thought on a bike, unless you want to end up head-over-heels on the side of the road, the only thing keeping you from a concussion being the helmet strapped to your chin.

And swimming, too, requires a certain attentiveness to breathing and staying afloat if you don't want to drown. While running, you can forget yourself, but in the pool, with the water splashing around your ears and into your eyes and nose, it's hard to go inside yourself in the same way.

It wasn't long after our move that my wife heard from a colleague about a yoga studio in town, and she began taking evening classes there. Aside from hiking in her youth, she'd never shown much interest in regular exercise before (except for a casual evening stroll after dinner or a walk on the beach), but now she had to acknowledge that she was getting older, too, and needed to find a way to stay in shape. Unexpectedly, she found the weekly yoga classes stimulating both physically and mentally. "You should try it," she told me each week after returning home from her class, still sweaty but glowing in a way that I'd never seen before. "It's relaxing."

Week after week she came home with that afterglow, and I began to notice how her posture changed. She now stood straighter, her shoulders pulled back, so she appeared taller. She became more limber, too, gaining the ability to peer over her shoulder with greater ease while driving rather than relying solely on her rearview mirrors before changing lanes. And she seemed calmer, less prone to rush, more willing to let life take its course and to follow it wherever it might lead. Curious about how these changes in her had come about and what might have drawn her into a daily commitment to yoga besides simply needing to stay in shape, I signed up for the next session's introductory class.

My class met on Wednesday evenings at the Garden of the Heart Yoga Center in a one-story, cinder-block building by the side of a small pond in one of Sarasota's industrial zones on the southeast side of town, a few miles from the famous white sand beaches of Siesta Key. I got into my car and drove the thirty minutes to the class, a bit anxious about what I was going to find. Would I feel out of place in a room full of women? Would I be able to do even the simplest of poses? Would I find yoga too foreign, as I'd feared years ago, too touchy-feely, for my taste?

I arrived at the center that first night thinking about these questions and wondering why I was so afraid of trying something new, worried about meeting new people, anxious about finding myself a student again, afraid of embarrassing myself. I was busy constructing obstacles and creating problems where none existed, except in my own mind. And I didn't even notice, half the time, that I was doing it.

That first night, I was so busy worrying about myself and how I'd feel in this unfamiliar setting that I didn't notice the sneakers and sandals lined up by the door when I walked into the center. Instead of removing my sneakers, I walked through the foyer and into the class, where other students were stretching and warming up, not quite sure where I was going or what I was supposed to do. It turned out to be my first yoga lesson: *pay attention!*

The other students were barefoot and already arranging blue rubber yoga mats on the floor, carefully setting blankets and belts and Styrofoam blocks nearby, along with water bottles and hand towels. Vesna, the instructor, a young woman with tanned arms, long, wavy black hair, and sparkling dark eyes, sat on her own mat, legs crossed, barefoot, in front of the *puja* table, which held a vase of fresh flowers and a thin stick of burning incense, reviewing her notes. She looked up in alarm when she saw me come into the room still wearing my sneakers. "No, no, no," she said gently, then rose and escorted me back to the foyer where she pointed at the shoes that I had passed by a few minutes earlier. "You must take off your shoes before entering."

Her voice was so kind, so soft, that I didn't take offense or feel embarrassed at my mistake. It was such a gentle rebuke, the way you might remind a child to finish a glass of milk before bedtime. I felt welcomed rather than scolded. I removed my sneakers and slipped them under the bench with the other footwear, leaving my socks on because I was embarrassed by the sight of my toenails. (Over the years, I had developed a bad case of fungus nail.) But, thank goodness, no one objected to my socks.

The rubber yoga mats were folded and stacked on shelves in the far corner of the room. I took one down and found a place along the rear wall, where I felt less visible than beside the students in the front row, closer to the teacher. Blankets, blocks, and belts were stored beside the mats, and I took one of each, not sure what I needed them for. I placed them between my mat and the wall, then sat down and tried not to stare too openly at the curves and rounded shapes—quite visible in the body-hugging shirts and pants—of the women stretching on either side of my mat.

We began class lying on our backs in Relaxation Pose, legs spread slightly, hands and arms relaxed at our sides. After six hours spent writing at my desk, I shut my eyes, stretched out my legs and arms, and listened to Vesna encourage us to let go of the day's problems and concerns, to return to our bodies, our breath, and allow ourselves to be present, in that moment. I let her voice seep into me. It felt almost like floating on a cloud or like wrapping myself in a warm blanket.

Like most people unfamiliar with yoga, I'd assumed it was simply an exercise program designed to reduce stress and improve flexibility. Little did I know that it was a collection of poses built around an ancient philosophy that helped you explore the very essence of human existence and learn how to live fully in each moment. All that I knew in those early sessions was that I trusted Vesna's voice as she led us into the poses. Her voice helped me notice the tiniest details of my breath, or how I might be unintentionally hunching my shoulders, or if my legs weren't positioned properly. Listening to her voice as we moved through the various poses, I felt calmer. And the anxiousness that had gripped my heart before those early sessions seemed to vanish, replaced by an inner calmness that I hadn't felt in years. By the end of each lesson, especially on that first night, I felt tears well up in my eyes. Somehow Vesna had helped me begin to shed the many masks that I wore to shield myself from the disappointments and challenges of life.

Each week I returned to my mat, closed my eyes, listened to Vesna's voice, and learned how to drop those masks to reveal and revel in my true self. I learned new poses week after week and, in exploring each new pose, learned how to trust my self. Over the next few weeks and months, as I learned a handful of new poses and noted how each pose sent a ripple effect of changes off the mat into my life, I watched as more and more of the shells that I had created to protect myself from the world fell away.

I learned how to let go of my ideas of perfection and worry less about failing. If I made a mistake, I learned how to let it go, the same way I learned to move on if I lost my balance in a pose. If I tried making a new friend, I learned to accept that it might not be my fault if the friendship didn't work out. And if I received feedback on a story that I'd sent out to friends or editors, I learned to welcome feedback without feeling hurt by the criticism.

With each Mountain Pose, I found myself standing straighter, taller. As I firmed my legs and drew my shoulders back, I heard Vesna's voice as she walked around the room, making sure that our poses were in alignment so we didn't hurt ourselves. And as I stood on my mat, feeling open to the world, prepared to welcome whatever challenges and disappointments life might still hold for me, I first began to hear the voice of my true self, the one I could trust, the one I'd been searching for all my life.

FROM MY JOURNAL

You're not who you think you are but something more. The hidden muscles that you awaken are signs of this hidden part of yourself, as well as reminders of the part of the world that is hidden, too, but which you can find if you search for it. Maybe what it means to find our balance is to find a way to link ourselves with the invisible source of energy that is at our core and at the core of life?

How did I learn to hear and trust my inner voice? It began, ironically, with a journal. As comfortable as I am with pen and paper—I've worked as a freelance writer or editor since graduating from college and kept a variety of journals with varying degrees of success—I never thought about keeping a practice journal until four years after that first yoga class. It was then that another teacher, Rita, gave each of us in her class a spiral-bound journal on the last day of our session together. "Give it a try," she said, pulling a journal out of the box and handing it to me. "See where it will lead you."

When I began keeping a journal to reflect on my yoga practice, the first thing that I needed to learn was how to listen to and trust the voice inside me, the voice that I'd first heard years ago when I'd kept a journal for my English professor in college, and which I'd rediscovered in the journals that I'd kept while my mother was dying of cancer. It was a voice that scared me because it made me feel so vulnerable and exposed, and yet that voice helped me feel more connected to myself—and to something larger than myself—than any other voice. If I was to fully understand myself and my relationship to the world and to others, I needed to find that voice again, to let go of my fear of being vulnerable and open. Rather, I needed to learn how to achieve the courage to be vulnerable and reveal more of myself to the world without fear of ridicule or criticism or disdain. It took writing pages and pages before I could let go of these fears and begin to hear my true voice and let it come through on the page. I could only detect that voice after I'd learned how to cast aside the voices of impersonators. I had to learn how to relax on the page, let down my defenses, and allow my heart to show in ways that I'd learned in my yoga classes over the past four years but hadn't yet incorporated into my daily life. I had to learn how to accept and let go of myself in order to be myself.

It wasn't easy. When you sit down to write something new, you face an empty page. You confront the fear that you may not have anything to say or, worse, that what you have to say may be unoriginal or foolish or downright stupid. I had to learn how to step into the silence of the page and trust that I wouldn't drown in silence, that the blank page wouldn't overwhelm me. For that to happen, I had to drop my defenses and reveal myself—not a caricature of myself, or an inflated image. I had to let myself show, warts and all. Anything less than complete honesty would have frightened my true voice and sent it skittering away in an instant.

In time, the combination of keeping a journal and practicing yoga helped me learn to view life in a nonjudgmental fashion, a neutral way that was altogether different than the way that I'd viewed the world in my youth, when I started keeping a personal journal. That earlier view was self-absorbed and turned inward. This view was focused on the relationship between the inner and outer worlds, viewing both simultaneously as places that can nurture growth if we can assume the proper attitude and perspective.

Keeping a journal has given me a way to find this perspective and to reflect on life. My journal is a safe place where I can ask questions, examine the sometimes confusing pieces that make up my life, and hear what I'm thinking and feeling when I can't always admit such thoughts or feelings aloud. On the page, I can explore in private whatever might trouble or excite or surprise me without fear of making mistakes or saying the wrong thing or appearing stupid or feeling invisible. (When I was younger, I felt as if every word written on the page in private were somehow being shouted to the world. Now, it feels like I'm whispering, and I'm the only one who can hear.)

In the pages of my journal, I don't have to try as hard as when I was younger. I don't need to change the world, merely accept it as it is. The page, just like the mat and the world itself, is neutral. It's like an empty vessel waiting to be filled, a blank slate yearning for words. The page offers no judgment or criticism. It's just paper, silently waiting for my pen, eager to reveal and let me hear my voice. It was this process of writing in the journal each day, before and after yoga practice, that helped me learn to lower my defenses, let go of the imposters and the fake voices, open up and write from my heart.

FROM MY JOURNAL

 Yoga—on the mat—is one place where I don't have to prove myself through my earning potential or productivity. It's a place where I can let down my guard and explore, for the sake of discovery, and not worry about the value others see in me, only the value that I perceive in myself. No, that's not right: the value of life for its own sake, living, breathing, as a way of celebrating all of life's possibilities.

In the beginning I worried the notebook might feel too much like work. But now I see it as a place to play and explore new ideas, the kind that don't usually appear when I'm perched at my desk instead of sitting cross-legged on my mat.

After mat: It's as if a strong wind has cleared out my mind's clutter. My worries are gone, replaced by clarity and sharpness of focus. Plus, there's a feeling of freedom. Images, memories, thoughts all flow in a random sequence . . . just flowing.

How can your journal help you accept the world and yourself in order to live more fully in each moment? Here are a few writing exercises to help you think about opening in new ways that you may find worth exploring.

Journal Practice: Opening Up

▸ Sit on your mat (or chair) in a comfortable position before you begin your yoga practice. Place your journal and a pen beside you. Adjust your position so you feel aligned and balanced. When you're ready to begin, close your eyes. Imagine that your body is a room and the poses that you are about to do serve as doorways into that room. Each pose, each open doorway, lets you see another side of that room, another side of yourself.

As you move from being seated into a pose, say Cat Tilt or Dog Tilt, keep your eyes closed, and look inside the room of your body. What do you see? Are muscles tense, resistant? Or are they relaxed and open? Again, as you move into the next pose, say the name of the pose to yourself—Downward-Facing Dog Pose or Mountain Pose—and ask yourself (with your eyes still shut) how the pose lets you see your body in a new light. When you're finished with your asana practice, fold into the Child's Pose—another doorway—and then move into Relaxation Pose. After a few minutes, sit up to end your practice.

Then pick up your journal and ask yourself what these poses, done with your eyes closed, helped you discover (or not) today. Write for at least five minutes.

➤ Before beginning your asana practice, sit on your mat in a comfortable position, your journal open in your lap, and consider what you want to explore through your practice. Do you want to look at your sense of impatience? Your search for balance? Your fear of letting yourself be too vulnerable? Your sense of isolation? Are you hesitant about making friends, taking risks, doing something for others, having fun? You can use your journal to explore any of these issues. Make notes in your journal about what you love and what frightens you, what you want most out of life and what you dread, whether you trust your friends and whether you think they can trust you.

Once you settle on a theme for your practice, a thread that you can weave from pose to pose, put your journal aside and begin your asana session. After you finish, pick up your journal again and write about how the poses helped (or distracted) you from exploring your theme. Did the journal help awaken you to new possibilities? How? And if not, why not? Write for at least five minutes.

➤ Find a comfortable seated position, either on your mat or in a chair. Close your eyes. Let your mind settle, drawing inward. Listen to the sounds around you, and eventually focus on the beating of your heart. Still your mind so you can hear your heart beating. Let yourself sink into that pulsating rhythm. Stay there for a while without moving, without worrying about what to think or what you think you should think. Just let your mind focus on your heartbeat. If your thoughts wander, gently bring them back to the rhythm of your heart. Notice your thoughts, let them go, notice, let go.

When you feel at ease and in rhythm with your heart, open your eyes. What's the first thing you see? Clouds outside your window? A stain on the ceiling? Dirty dishes in the sink? It might be the carpet, or a picture on a wall, or someone walking past your window. Open your journal, pick up your pen, and write down what you see. Then close your eyes again, and focus on your heart's rhythm. How has your experience changed? Contrast the way you see the world with your eyes open and your eyes closed. What thoughts or feelings arise with your eyes open? With your eyes closed? Write for at least ten minutes.

2: Moving Past Fear

So many worries . . . and none of the worries
really matter in the end, do they? I can only
accomplish what my body will let me do today.
—FROM MY JOURNAL

It sounds foolish now, but I almost didn't enroll in Rita's class. That's because her class was scheduled to meet on Tuesday mornings, from 10 to 11:30, unlike my class with Jaye, which I'd been taking for the past few sessions, and which met early on Thursday mornings, from 8 to 9:30. The earlier time slot gave me a chance to fit in a morning's writing and editing after class, once I got back home. Switching to Rita's later class would mean losing the morning hours before noon for work, the time of day when I felt the most productive. With my other obligations— picking up my daughter at school every afternoon at 4, stopping at the supermarket to buy groceries, cleaning the house, preparing dinner—I was worried that I wouldn't be able to make up the lost time.

On one hand, the class on Thursdays served as an informal coda for the week, a comforting way of reminding myself of all that I'd accomplished since the start of the week on Monday and reinvigorating me as I looked at the remainder of the week. Coming to class on Thursdays was a bit like reaching the top of a hill. I could look back on the distance that I'd come over the week and, at the same time, gaze ahead to where I still had to go. It gave a certain rhythm to my week. I didn't want to lose that rhythm, that sense of progress, as I worked on various projects.

On the other hand, Nicole, one of my friends in the class, had announced that she was eager to move up to the next level, excited about beginning the inversions—Headstands and Handstands—that the students in Rita's class were working on. Everything we had learned in our class with Jaye had prepared her for this step forward into the upside-down world of inversions, and she couldn't wait to get started. But I didn't share her enthusiasm. The last time I could remember doing a handstand was in fifth grade, when I tumbled head over heels on the grass, never quite able to keep myself aloft. So I wasn't looking forward to learning inversions that might lead to injury, the very thing that I'd tried to avoid by beginning yoga. If you want to know the truth, I was more than a little frightened by the idea of going upside down. But my fear had nothing to do with physical limitations, which shouldn't be ignored when deciding to do a pose; rather, it had to do with psychological limits that I had created to keep myself "safe" from perceived harm or failure. Did I truly need such limits to keep me safe? Or was I simply creating unnecessary boundaries for myself out of fear?

But Jaye gently encouraged me to move up to Rita's class. He shrugged off my concerns and literally pushed me out the door, the way a mother bird might shove her fledgling out of the nest. "You'll be fine," he said, confident that I could fly on my own, having taught me all that I needed to know to take the next step.

Jaye might have believed that I could handle the demands of the next level, but I knew that I hadn't yet mastered all the poses in his class—not that anyone ever really "masters" any of the poses. But there were still plenty of asanas for me to learn and refine, especially back bends, poses that I found excruciatingly difficult because of the stiffness in my upper back, the result, most likely, of spending hours hunched over my desk.

Even so, I told myself, maybe it wasn't fear that kept me from moving to the next level. Maybe I had settled into a comfort zone, and it was simply laziness, not wanting to push myself. Or maybe it was knowing what I could do and not wanting to explore new territory. Did this reluctance to explore new things equal fear? I wasn't sure. I didn't want to think of myself as a coward, but maybe I was, too ashamed to admit my fears.

FROM MY JOURNAL

A low, gray sky brings rain for the first time in weeks. It's chilly (for April)—high sixties. I'm thinking how I hold onto each day, not wanting to let go, unwilling to let the days pass. It's as if I'm afraid life will evaporate in front of my eyes.

On the drive home after one of my Thursday classes with Jaye, I asked myself if perhaps I had come to rely too much on Jaye and his teaching methods. A slim, graceful man in his early forties, Jaye's energy seemed boundless as he led us through the various poses with a deceptive ease, making clear a new or difficult pose whenever he saw confusion on our faces. Throughout the class, especially at the start, when we gathered in a circle, he offered bits of wisdom from his well of experiences or from his classes with John Friend, founder of Anusara Yoga.

Jaye's lessons at the start of each class were often filled with a dry wit, a remnant of his British ancestry, perhaps, and his classes were challenging and fun and always exhausting. In his younger years, he had trained as a dancer with the Joffrey Ballet, in New York, and on some days he could assume, albeit unintentionally, a slightly authoritarian tone that was hard for me to hear because of my own tendency to judge myself too critically

Even though he was gentle and unassuming, and his lessons were filled with the wisdom he'd acquired from years of studying the body and its movements, he communicated high expectations to his students as we entered each pose. And when he demonstrated a pose, I felt as if he expected us to follow the movements into the pose so precisely that it could feel as if I were learning to do Jaye's pose rather than exploring my own pose. That was my way of hearing his instructions. I'd begun to wonder if learning the pose as Jaye wanted us to do it might limit the way I might do the pose on my own.

And yet, even with such questions, I didn't want to think about leaving his class. I'd grown to love the stories with which he opened each class—self-deprecating stories about a getting lost driving to the grocery store, humorous tales about efforts that didn't pan out, inspiring stories about his garden—an English-style garden in southwest Florida—or about students he'd met in his travels as a yoga teacher, stories of courage and faith and dedication. All the stories were told in his gentle voice, as if he were speaking directly to each of us, as if each student were the only person in the room and he had all the time in the world.

I admired his attention to detail and the way he talked us through each pose, pointing out the safe way to enter into the pose and the dangerous way, showing us the physics of each pose, the way an architect might describe a bridge or building, explaining why it worked and why it was effective and how it would benefit us. His understanding of the body and its muscles and organs, how everything was interrelated and how each part could impact other parts, was phenomenal. How could I leave this world that I knew for a world that was unknown?

The only thing that I'd heard about Rita's class, aside from Nicole's excitement, was what another student in Jaye's class told me one morning. "We spent a lot of time upside down," Ed said, as he stretched on the mat next to mine, warming up in preparation for our Thursday morning class. "Too much time for me. That's why I came back to Jaye." Ed was more than a few years older than me, a kind man in his sixties with striking white hair and a trim body that gave him the appearance of a man twenty years younger. In class we offered encouragement to one another whenever Jaye asked us to stretch ourselves into a demanding position. Maybe he simply was too old to do inversions, I told myself, and I shouldn't pay attention. Or maybe he has a point, and I should follow his lead. What's the sense, after all, of spending so much time upside down, when our entire lives are spent right side up?

So I listened to my doubts, rationalized my worries, and surrendered to my hesitancy, my fear. I didn't move up to Rita's class that session. I wasn't ready. Instead, I remained in Jaye's class, comforted by Ed's presence on the mat next to mine. It didn't matter that I'd explored most of the poses in previous sessions. What mattered, I thought at the time, was that I had found a way to settle and calm myself, leave behind the worries and anxieties of my work—always wrapped up in words, tense, uncertain—and escape from the troubles that were waiting for me back at my desk.

But I listened closely to the reports my wife shared each week after her class with Rita. She had signed up for two classes a week that session, one with Rita on Tuesday mornings, the other with Jaye on Thursday mornings. She loved both of them. By the end of the next session, I'd decided to push past my fear of the unknown and make the break from Jaye. After more than four sessions—almost two years—in his class, I felt that I'd started to repeat myself, covering ground that I'd already explored. I no longer felt that I was challenging myself to grow and expand, and a different kind of fear—fear of stagnation—propelled me forward.

I would miss Ed's comforting presence. I would miss Jaye's stories. But at the start of the next session, I went ahead and signed up for Rita's class on Tuesday mornings. What did I have to lose, really? If I didn't enjoy her more advanced class, or if I found that I had trouble with the inversions, I could always return to Jaye's class and find a place waiting for me.

FROM MY JOURNAL

Fear can rob you of life, I tell myself, if you let it control your thoughts, your actions. How does yoga help conquer fear? Maybe it helps us face reality? In each pose, if I breathe deeply into pain, perhaps I can pass through it? Maybe it helps us see pain as part of life rather than as part of life to be denied? I don't know. Maybe not all the answers can be found on the mat.

After mat: Sunlight gleams on green leaves. The sky is deep blue. Spanish moss tendrils spin in the breeze.

Stepping into Rita's class the first time took a bit of an adjustment, both mentally and physically. The room was located on the opposite side of the reception area from Jaye's classroom, and it was much smaller and narrower than the wider room where we met for Jaye's classes. A large window on the north wall overlooked a small pond, and another, smaller window faced the parking lot to the west. But even with the windows, the room still felt extremely close, especially after we rolled out our mats, only a few inches separating us from each other instead of the few feet of separation that I'd come to expect in Jaye's class. And the room heated up quickly, even with the air conditioning on high, as soon as we started working hard at the poses, although there were only a dozen of us. But it wasn't the size of the room that I found most challenging. It was Rita herself. A tall, striking woman without an ounce of fat to hide her bones, she radiated an intense energy and passion when she welcomed us into the room. Unlike Jaye's classes, which were relatively calm and quiet before we began each week's lesson, each student finding his or her way to the mat and warming up in silence, Rita's classes were alive with the bubbly sounds of student voices mixing with her own exclamations of surprise or squeals of welcome each time another person entered the room.

Joining her students as they set up their mats that morning, I felt a certain camaraderie, a lighthearted playfulness, that was new to me, as if I'd stepped into a women's locker room or had joined a dance class before the start of rehearsal. Voices crisscrossed the room. Friends embraced each other, and Rita joined in a group hug. News of the week—a child's illness, a husband's travel plans, a book or movie recommendation—was exchanged as we warmed up on our mats.

Jaye's classes were always challenging and often fun, but I wouldn't describe them as playful or as loosely structured as Rita's classes. In Jaye's classes, which were meticulously organized, we rarely deviated from the plan that he'd prepared for the class. In Rita's, it felt like just the opposite because she was always willing to explore different questions and to follow them wherever they might lead. Her flexible approach to the day's plan helped me begin to understand that there were different ways of practicing yoga, even within the same studio, and that a pose could be explored from more than one viewpoint. Her lessons were the epitome of playfulness, even as we struggled to learn new and challenging poses, and the playfulness helped us all loosen up a little and explore the poses without worrying about how we looked. Instead, we could enjoy the process of discovering the pose.

It took a number of weeks for me to feel comfortable with the lively chatter that filled the room throughout the class. I was stunned by the steady stream of questions back and forth from student to student as we held each pose, and from students to Rita, and from Rita back to the students. I was accustomed to hearing only one voice—Jaye's—in class, and to exploring each pose in silence, as I tried to pay attention to what my various muscles were or weren't able to do.

But soon the questioning and the casual banter made each pose feel like a new journey, both personal and communal, and I began to feel myself loosening up a little more each week. Little by little, I found that I could take greater and greater risks, pushing myself past my fear a little further. No longer was I trying to model my pose on an ideal image that I held. I found with Rita's assistance that I could investigate the pose in a way that would make it my own. I left her class in amazement each week, feeling that I had reached a new level of understanding in my practice. Who knew you could laugh and play while learning yoga?

I stopped feeling as if I were pushing myself. With Rita's encouragement, I could relax into a pose instead of trying to force myself into it. Yes, I missed Jaye's stories. And I missed even more, especially in those first weeks, the sense of security that Jaye gave each student. He taught a pose in such a way that when you tried it yourself you felt protected by an invisible safety net that he had spread beneath you to catch you if you fell.

In Rita's class, there was no net. Instead, we supported each other during challenging poses by offering encouragement or gentle jokes or a kind remark. In Rita's class we became the net for each other, the *kula,* or community, that Rita helped us form. And, in the process of becoming part of the net, the kula, I found that I no longer feared falling or—more important— failing. Even so, I was anxious each time I stepped into Rita's class, unsure of what to expect. It felt just like when I'd started taking yoga classes.

But this uncertainty, this new fear, was an unexpected gift. It forced me to look deeper inside myself for support. Each time I felt anxious or nervous, I had to listen harder to my inner voice— the one that was warning me to be careful, suggesting that I might be taking too great a risk—and evaluate it. Was it telling me the truth? Or was it simply expressing my fears—fear of the unknown, fear of making a mistake, fear of looking foolish, fear of failing? Where was this voice coming from, I wondered? What was I supposed to make of it? And could I find a way to simply listen to it without judging it one way or another?

It took weeks and weeks and a good deal of patience (more than I thought I possessed) to learn how to listen to that voice. I call it my alarmist's voice, a voice that would warn me of the dangers that I was facing in each new pose, especially when we began to explore handstands. Going upside down was disorienting. Each time we prepared to do Handstand, I could hear the voice gaining strength and could feel the knot of fear tighten in my stomach.

I was frightened that something might happen once I went upside down, that I'd have a brain aneurysm or something equally catastrophic. Seriously. I even tried to mask my fear by joking about it with the class. They thought the idea of a brain aneurysm was outrageous. Most of the students in the class groaned, but some laughed while kicking up into Handstand. Not me. I wasn't laughing. I was too nervous, too worried, too busy listening to that voice of alarm warning me to be careful. Too busy trying to get past my own fear.

Unexpectedly, I found the sympathetic responses of the rest of the class comforting. If they thought my fears were unfounded and truly outrageous, perhaps I was simply overreacting in the way that I'm prone to overdramatize a difficult situation. And with their support I managed to push away my fears and kick into Handstand and hold the pose for longer than I'd expected.

FROM MY JOURNAL

On my way to class, I imagine Handstand as an insurmountable mountain, a challenge—like a huge boulder—standing in my path. I feel anxious entering class, not really relaxed. Maybe it's because I'm uncomfortable with the idea of failing or making a mistake or not being able to do what the other students can do?

I try to visualize myself going into a Handstand, and then Rita tells us about the class's theme—freedom: how you establish freedom in yoga by creating space. Hearing her talk about space somehow gives me the room to explore Handstand, to see it not as an impediment to somewhere else but as a path in itself. And when the time comes for Handstand, I pull my mat to the wall, set my foundation in Downward-Facing Dog Pose, and through some magic kick up into Handstand.

I can't say what's different from last week. Maybe my arms are farther apart. Or maybe I position my hands farther away from the wall. Or maybe I can "see" myself going up. Whatever the reason, I swing up—feet against the wall—into Handstand and hold the pose until I lower my legs slowly—one at a time—to come back to earth.

JOURNAL PRACTICE: MOVING PAST FEAR

» What are you afraid of? Pain? Loneliness? Failure? Loss? Success? Sit on your mat, or wherever you feel most comfortable, and make a list of the ten things that you're most fearful of. Here's my list: (1) fear of heights, (2) fear of rejection, (3) fear of intimacy, (4) fear of failure, (5) fear of letting go of those I love, (6) fear of embarrassment, (7) fear of getting older, (8) fear of dying, (9) fear of not living life fully in each moment, (10) fear of losing my memory and my ability to write.

Once you've created your list, sit with it, study each item carefully, and notice your response to it. Does your stomach clench? Does your jaw tighten? Do your palms start to itch and sweat? When you find the item that intensifies the fear that you feel in the pit of your stomach, write it down at the top of a blank page in your journal. Ask yourself why it makes you feel afraid. Then spend five minutes writing about what you most fear and why you think it's so unsettling. If you feel comfortable reviewing what you've written, take a few moments to reread your words and notice any change in your body's sensations, in your response to whatever you may fear.

▸ Write about an incident in your life when you felt intensely frightened—not simply mild anxiety or a heightened sense of danger but the dry-mouth, knuckle-clenching kind of fear that makes you want to bolt from your seat. Take a few moments to reimagine the event. Set the scene leading up to the event without entering the event itself. Just follow the steps up to the event as if you were climbing the stairway to a closed door. And do the same for the scene leading away from the event when you felt safe again, when you could still feel the fear but no longer felt threatened by it. When you're ready, go back to the scene leading up to the event, and climb the stairs again to that closed door. Reach out and turn the doorknob. Push open the door. Go back into the event that frightened you. Can you stay with it and describe it (as if you were a camera lens filming the event from a place on the wall)? Can you step through the event from beginning to end and move past your fear? If so, describe how you were able to go beyond your fear. If not, describe what happened to keep you from moving past your fear. If writing about this incident heightens fear or anxiety, put down your pen, close your journal, and return to the sound of your breath. Listen to your heart beating. Remind yourself that you are here now and are safe.

▸ Fear can become a roadblock, an obstacle, a speed bump that makes it difficult for you to move forward. How can you move past fear? If you have a fear of heights, for example, how do you manage to drive over bridges, or step into elevators, or climb mountains? Can you describe your fear by giving an example of when you felt it most intensely? What sensations do you remember? And can you write about how you might move past or around your fear? If you find that you can't move past or around your fear—if, for example, you can't overcome your fear of bridges—you need to learn how to live with your fear. (That may mean taking a longer route, perhaps, to avoid the bridge and reaching your destination a little later.) In writing about your fears, you may discover the very path that will take you past them.

3: Accepting Gifts

Can you find a way, within the heat, to feel cool?
Can you find a way to look at the sunlight and see shadows?
—FROM MY JOURNAL

It was due to Rita's gracious manner that the class came together. She invited her students to share themselves without any preconditions, and we felt this openness immediately. Not only did she hug students when they arrived in her class, she stopped whatever she was doing to check in with new arrivals. And she unflinchingly shared parts of her own life—the difficulties that she had getting out of the house that morning, the challenges with traffic on the way to the studio—in ways that made her less imposing as a teacher, almost like a friend, which is what she had become to many in the class.

She understood each of the poses on a deep level, as if she'd absorbed them into her sinews and bones, and she could skillfully demonstrate why someone might be having a problem. Unlike Jaye, who defined the poses with such precision, Rita didn't always need words. Sometimes she simply came over and made an adjustment in a student's pose without uttering a word. And the student would realign her pose and suddenly understand it in her sinews and bones, too. It was magical, a form of teaching that was new to me and one that, at times, made me feel confused by my lack of knowledge.

In her opening comments to the class each week, Rita would invite us to gather around her in a circle and set an intention or theme for the class to focus on. But I didn't always understand what she was getting at, mystified by the references to Sanskrit sources. Rita's knowledge of yoga's history and philosophy was so profound that sometimes I felt like a beginner in an advanced-level class, unable to grasp the new ways she was suggesting to look at a pose or at life. And I felt most lost when, during these sessions, she turned the questions back on her students and asked each of us to speak instead of her. But this very process of being asked to step outside my comfort zone ultimately helped me feel less invisible in class. I started to learn, thanks to Rita's way of teaching (which relied on the student as much as the teacher), how to look inside myself—past my fear—for the kind of security and insights into the poses that I thought only a teacher like Jaye could provide.

FROM MY JOURNAL

I don't know what kind of practice will unfold today. If I try to make more room, more spaciousness, will that merely open myself up to more anger, more disappointment, more frustration?

Will it only open the floodgates of past failures, and the emotions attendant on them, rather than make space for new ways of seeing the world?

Spaciousness isn't only about making space, evidently. It's about learning what to place—and how to arrange —whatever you place in your newfound space.

After mat: In trying to make more spaciousness, I focused on the space between my fingers and toes—and from there to my lungs and heart—and realized you could easily fill the space newly created with thoughts of kindness and gratitude, compassion and community. You can choose whatever suits you to fill your space.

Every week, arriving early at the center, I unrolled my mat in the northwest corner of the class at the front of the room. That way, I was able to face the front window and look out over the lake during our asana practice. Next to me, Nicole set up her mat. And behind me was Jeanne, and next to her, Lena and Pat. Others found their places in the room, too: Anita, Carolyn, Kathy, Sandy, Phyllis, Debbi, Mary, and students who dropped in or wanted to make up a class. Each student had a special relationship with Rita. With everyone she seemed able to pick up the conversation as if she'd just spoken with them minutes earlier, rather than not having seen them for weeks or months.

Rarely did Rita play music in class. There was just the sound of her voice as she led us through the poses, or asked various students how they felt in a pose or what they'd done over the weekend, or described her own adventures on long bike rides that she took with her partner to raise money for MS or other causes. She lived in St. Petersburg, where she taught another yoga class, and commuted to Chicago once a month to lead yoga classes there, too, in addition to teaching in Sarasota. She was busy, and she shared with us how hectic her life felt sometimes. But even though her life outside class might have seemed chaotic, the moment the class started, she was present, utterly focused on the lesson and on her students, and nothing outside the class mattered—only this pose, this moment. We didn't need music. Rita's spirit seemed to sing to us during the ninety minutes that we spent with her.

I can't explain how it happened, but somehow, in some mysterious and gentle way, Rita drew me out of the shell of fear that I'd hidden in for years. It was a shell that I wasn't even aware of until I'd shed it. Of course, it's possible that yoga itself helped me begin the process of coming out of my shell. Perhaps it was only in Rita's class that I became aware of it and could reflect on the process with greater understanding.

But it wasn't only Rita who helped me. It was the class itself, the *kula*, as Rita called it, the other students surrounding me, the way the women interacted with each other, sharing weekly high points in their lives or laughing over a silly comment or boosting each other's spirits if someone was going through a difficult time—a broken foot, a divorce, the death of a younger sister, the loss of a dear aunt.

After our first few sessions together, most of the women, all roughly in their forties and fifties, some slightly older, some slightly younger, reached out to include me in their circle. It was as if, by working our bodies through the series of poses that Rita had planned for us each Tuesday morning, we could forget our bodies—the maleness of mine, the femaleness of theirs— and share the essence of our lives, heart to heart, reaching out from mat to mat within that small room to embrace one another as we struggled with Headstand for the first time or tried to move into a difficult twist. Maybe it was Rita's sense of playfulness that allowed us all to open up. Or maybe it was simply the unusual chemistry in that class, where everyone seemed to like and respect one another.

I don't recall how word got out that I was a writer and editor, but before long Rita began to turn to me during class to help refine her description of an idea or a pose. Her requests surprised me, took me out of my introverted, quiet shyness. She asked me to *think* about the poses. Not only did her questions prompt me to consider how a pose might make me feel, but they led to new insights about life, about how I might relate to myself on the mat and others off the mat, and to begin sharing these insights with the class. Even before giving me the journal, Rita helped me in her thoughtful, subtle way begin the process of reflection that led to writing in my journal and, ultimately, to this book. (Looking back on these classes from the distance of a few years, I can see how Rita designed the questions to draw me and the other students out of our shells, not because she needed any help.)

In Jaye's classes, the questions he asked were mostly rhetorical, intended to stimulate his students to think about the poses within the context of our yoga practice (or maybe he expected answers that I wasn't yet ready to give). What are the five basic principles of Anusara Yoga? Can you define inner spiral in a given pose? But Rita's questions were different; she asked them wanting answers. And knowing that she wanted an answer forced me to step outside the experience on the mat, put my body on "pause," so to speak, and think about her questions with my mind, not just my body. Unexpectedly, I found myself searching for the right words to describe an experience that until that moment had been wordless. And I learned to share the words with the class.

It wasn't easy at first. I had to think rather than let my mind wander in the sensations of the poses. I wasn't accustomed to using words in yoga, where so much of the pleasure for me was the nonverbal nature of the practice. In fact, it was the wordless nature of yoga that had drawn me so strongly to it initially. So much of my day is spent immersed in words, searching for the "right" word. When I first stepped onto a yoga mat and was given permission to let go of words, release the stresses and strains of my day, and notice instead the feelings beneath the words, I could relax the muscles and bones and sinews out of which the words flowed, and I felt enormous relief.

FROM MY JOURNAL

If I blur my vision, closing my eyes to squint, the black mat beneath me looks like the night sky. I feel as if I'm floating through space, or suspended, breathing in, breathing out, part of the solar system, a star shining bright in the galaxy.

When I open my eyes and look up, I see sunlight slanting across the back yard. I hear the breeze in the trees and the crunch of leaves beneath the paws of an animal—a raccoon or possum, a squirrel, a cat, a fox—as mysterious as the sound of the wind.

My muscles are stiff after two days of bicycling hard. They shout to be stretched and made flexible again. They seek limberness instead of strength, balance instead of forward motion. They seek a state of suspension where they can float. I want to feel all my senses at work. I don't want to go anywhere. I just want to stand in one place, being.

Until I'd come to yoga and lay down on the mat, I had never experienced such a release from the self-critical voice that berated me for failing to find a story line or for not revising a sentence or paragraph properly the first time. It was thanks to my first teacher, Vesna, that I had come to see yoga as a refuge from words while, at the same time, it helped me begin the search for my voice, for words that emerged from my heart, not just my head. Little by little, Vesna had guided us to a place that was far from words, and, in the process, she had guided me to the source of words. She asked us to let our toes relax while we lay in Relaxation Pose and to let our feet drop with gravity and to continue letting go of the tension—knees, thighs, hips, heart, all the way up to lips and eyes—until we reached a kind of bliss, undisturbed by the troubles or challenges or obstacles in our lives. Simply at rest. Breathing.

Only when we arrived in that place would our class begin. That was my introduction to yoga: Vesna's voice. Her encouragement to notice the details of our body's responses—how our lips pressed firmly together, how the tongue lightly touched the roof of the mouth, how we might clench our fists or feel tension in our eyes. Relax the skin, Vesna would say. Let gravity pull you into the earth. Let your breath wash away all stress. It was such a moving, wordless experience that first time, feeling my body without being critical, without judging or being judged, without having to translate my thoughts or sensations into words. It was so miraculous, so different from what I experienced in my everyday life. It was like meeting a long-lost friend.

Each class after that first session with Vesna, whether it was Nancy's or Cory's or Jaye's, helped me peel away the layers of resentment, fear, and disappointment that were keeping me from enjoying my life in the way that I hadn't enjoyed it since childhood. It was as if my daily concerns about writing had created a misalignment in my approach to words, and yoga was helping me find the proper alignment again. Each class led to a new view of myself, a new understanding of my voice.

Vesna's gentleness, Cory's precision in describing poses, Nancy's exploration of energy in "passive" poses, Jaye's drive for the truth, the essence, of a pose, and Rita's openness and playfulness: each showed me how to reconnect with parts of myself that I'd lost touch with over the years. But it was in Rita's class that I felt as if I'd shed a cloak that I hadn't even known I was wearing. It was as if I'd been hiding unbeknownst to myself behind an invisible screen. In Rita's class that screen dissolved.

At the end of the spring session, before we left for a week-long break from classes, Rita went into the kitchen, where everyone put their purses and sweaters and car keys, and she returned with a big brown cardboard box filled with spiral journals. Handing a journal to each of us, Rita explained that she kept journals, lots of journals, and that she hoped these would help us develop our own practice at home, help us deepen our understanding of the poses and our relationship to them.

The journal was slightly larger than my hand, with lined, cream-colored pages (blank on the back), a black spiral binding, and a cover, both front and back, wrapped in cloth on which was reproduced a Japanese painting—Katsushika Hokusai's "The Great Wave Off Kanagawa"—depicting a tall blue ocean wave frozen at its crest, just before it falls back to earth. In the distance, beneath the curl of the wave's white crest, you could see a snow-covered mountain. And entering the picture from the right-hand side you could make out the prows of two wooden vessels, coming from no one knows where and whose destination is also a mystery.

It was a beautiful gift, a hundred blank pages waiting for words (and pictures) to fill them, and I held it in my hand as the other students began rolling up their mats. I was mesmerized by the painting on the cover, the sense of power of the sea, and the two boats with their unknown passengers and captains, sailing into a mystery. The picture seemed like the perfect metaphor for our lives. All of us are caught in the curl of a wave, our passage from birth to death a mystery. All we can know (like the passengers on the boats) is this moment, and the next, and the next. I mentioned this to Rita, who gave me a hug in response, and said, when I asked her what I should write, "Let it take you somewhere." In that moment, the journal became one of the boats in the painting, a craft carrying me across the sea toward a destination that I still don't know but that I keep sailing toward, moment by moment.

As I left the class that day, unsure if the journal simply meant more work or if it would lead me to something else, I heard Rita's voice encouraging me to take the risk. In the end, I had to trust that the laws of nature and the forces of the universe would lead me where I needed to go. Trust, as it turned out, was part of the gift that Rita gave me.

FROM MY JOURNAL

 *Today is the first time I'm writing in the journal that Rita gave us. I'm sitting cross-legged on my mat, outside, by the pool. It's quiet. But in the quiet I hear the thrumming of an airplane's engine, the hum of a neighbor's air conditioner, the call of a bird—*cheep, cheep, cheep—*deep in the woods, the buzz of insects—crickets or cicadas, perhaps. But, mostly, I hear the incessant call of that one bird.*

The temperature has risen to eighty degrees. The air is so soft you don't feel it on the surface of your skin, except when

the breeze blows, like now, gently, rustling the palm fronds. And then the return of the bird's call. Maybe that bird's call is what I need to hear today. Maybe it's the spirit of the bird—calling to its mate, announcing its presence, or singing of the glory of life—that I honor with my practice today.

After mat: Utter stillness when I rise from my last pose: Relaxation Pose. No wind. No jet engines. No air conditioner pumps. Just silence. Even the bird is silent.

JOURNAL PRACTICE: ACCEPTING GIFTS

▸ Sitting comfortably on your mat, close your eyes and recall a special gift that you've received. What makes the gift special? Without lifting your pen or opening your journal, keep your eyes closed and imagine the gift and the moment that you accepted it. Try to remember how you felt at that moment. When you've got a clear picture of that moment in your mind, open your eyes, pick up your pen, turn to a blank page in your journal, and begin writing. Describe the gift in detail. Do you recall the physical sensations that you felt when you received it? Were your hands hot or cold? Was your pulse racing? And how did it change or deepen your relationship with the source of the gift? And, last, how did it change the way you view yourself and your relationship to the world? Write for ten minutes or more.

- With your journal open and your pen ready to start writing, make a list of the gifts in your life. Then select two of the gifts—the one that you feel has had the most impact on your life and the one that you feel has had little impact—and compare the two. Is the one as important or the other as insignificant as you may think? What do these gifts have in common? And how do they differ? And do you appreciate each in different ways after writing about them?

- As you begin your asana practice, think of each pose, and each pause between poses, as a gift. How does each gift change the way you see the world? Notice how each gift leads to another, and another, each one altering your way of being in the world. When you've finished your practice, take a few moments to collect your thoughts on what it means to receive a gift and how a gift can change your life. Ask yourself if you're open to change, no matter how small the change may prove to be.

- Write about welcoming life's changes as gifts. For example, if you find it difficult to accept gifts, write about why you find it hard. Or, if you love receiving gifts, write about what it is about a gift that makes you feel special. Write about how being receptive to life's offerings impacts your life. Write about how you can take steps in your asana practice, in your life, to encourage yourself to be receptive, accepting. Examine the obstacles (critical voices, fears, mistrust of others or of yourself) that might stand in the way.

4: Paying Attention

My mind is an observer, monitoring my breath,
my stretches, my balance. It's like an inner 'eye,' always
watching, not judging, simply observing: this, then that.
—FROM MY JOURNAL

Over time, through practicing yoga and keeping a journal, I learned that the destination wasn't as important as the process. What do you notice in this moment? What do you notice now? Using a journal, keeping a record of what I came to notice day after day, even if I didn't reread what I'd written, helped me pay closer attention to my life. I began to notice changes, microscopic changes at first, then larger changes, as a result of my practice.

That first time I entered the yoga studio, when I'd made the mistake of not removing my shoes, I hadn't seen the shoes and sandals by the door. I hadn't known that we were expected to remove our footwear before stepping into the room. I had felt so embarrassed. Why hadn't I noticed that everyone else but me was walking barefoot in the studio? I went back and kicked off my sneakers, but I didn't want to remove my socks. Something about revealing my feet made me feel exposed and vulnerable.

I don't know about your feet, but I'm convinced that my feet are ugly because eight of the ten nails are discolored by fungus. I have no idea how I developed fungus nail—some say that runners, with the heavy pounding that their feet have to endure, are more prone to fungus nail than others. The condition isn't painful, just unsightly, and I feel embarrassed that I don't have more normal-looking feet. It doesn't help matters that the little toe on each foot is barely developed, the tiny nail almost invisible.

It's not that I don't like my feet. I've run hundreds of miles thanks to my feet and have walked hundreds more, so I have a special affection for them. I've soaked them in Epsom salts, I've treated their blisters and sores after races, and I've rubbed ice over my heels when tendinitis made running excruciatingly painful. But as much as I love my feet, I'm ashamed of the way they look, embarrassed that they don't appear stronger, perhaps more masculine. (My mother's feet had the same tiny little toe.) So, I don't walk around barefoot (except on the beach) or wear sandals. As far as I'm concerned, my feet are a part of my body that I don't want to have much contact with. So, for that first class, I left my socks on, which was fine with Vesna. And although the soles of my feet slipped a little on the mat, I didn't have any trouble with the poses.

But some time during the session I began to wonder what it would feel like to remove my socks and walk barefoot across the floor like the other students and feel the mat without it slipping beneath my feet. In the evening, after class, I would stare down at my feet in the shower at home and wonder. Maybe they aren't so ugly after all. Maybe they are my feet, not an imposter's. That tiny little toe—so what if my mom had the same tiny toe? That didn't mean I had her feet. They were mine, and maybe I could try to appreciate the way that tiny toe linked me to my mother instead of resenting it for being like hers. Maybe I didn't have to judge my feet as ugly or beautiful or boring or pale. Maybe I didn't have to compare my feet—or me—to anything else. They were simply feet. Everybody has them.

So, the following week, I sat down on the bench in the foyer, took off my sneakers, and slowly removed my socks before class. I wiggled my toes in the air. I pressed my bare soles into the floor. For the first time in years I paid attention to my feet and felt free, the way you feel when you walk across a beach. I looked down at my feet as we stood in Mountain Pose to begin the class. I stretched out my toes (all except that pinky toe, which just hangs there). I rooted the four corners of each foot into the ground. I could feel the earth supporting me, could feel the direct connection to the earth through the flesh on the soles of my feet.

Barefoot, I came into Downward-Facing Dog Pose and could grip the mat with my toes. In Relaxation Pose, I could feel the breeze from the air conditioning blowing on my feet. After a few more sessions, I didn't even notice that I was going barefoot, and no one else noticed either. No one stared at my feet. No one commented on my fungus nails. No one pointed and laughed at my little toe. I felt like a child again, running barefoot through the grass.

When I reflected on that early experience in my yoga practice and wrote about it a few years later in my journal, I could remember and understand it at the same time. Writing in my journal lets me revisit the events of the past and see what I might have missed at the time or gain a new understanding of what took place. The process of writing lets me examine the things I may have an aversion toward, as well as the things I may be attracted to, in a neutral setting, so I can examine the aversion or attraction without losing myself in the emotion of the moment. The journal's page provides distance and gives me a new perspective. With pen in hand, I can observe myself and pay attention to my responses in a way that sheds light on how I act and why. The new perspective can help me choose different ways of acting in the future.

If you like the feel of bare feet on the floor, for instance, you can rediscover that joy in the pages of your journal and remind yourself to go barefoot more often. If you enjoy sitting on your mat, then sit on it! The first time I sat on my mat in that first class long ago, I remember how surprised I was by the shift in perspective, how the world and my view of it changed when I lowered myself to the ground. No longer was I commanding a view of the world from six feet in the air. Only three feet above the surface, I felt as if I'd gained a new understanding of the way I had been inhabiting the world, walking through it without really seeing or noticing it.

On the floor, I felt more closely linked to the earth, could feel it spinning beneath me, sending out waves of energy. I could roll and lie down and play in ways that I hadn't played since childhood. Something about sitting on the floor released my inhibitions. On the floor, I could be myself; I could relax in the prone position and let my muscles loosen and feel the bones drop and know the earth beneath my bones would hold me up. That sense of unconditional support and shared energy was a new feeling. By letting go of my socks and walking barefoot onto the mat, I found a different way of being.

FROM MY JOURNAL

While doing yoga poses, I feel like a blank slate and simply let impressions of sight and touch fall like chalk dust on the slate. I don't erase or add. I simply let the impressions fall on the slate, indiscriminately, without judging them.

This rhythm feels like a series of consecutive waves coming toward shore that I don't want to miss. I wait for each wave to lift me up, to show me the arc of my breath, the spray of my thoughts, the mystery of how I am linked through thoughts and breath to others and to something larger than all of us.

Sometimes I think yoga is about finding the link to this force, this energy, and reaffirming its existence in the universe and our link to it. It's a kind of prayer.

Each class brought a new insight, a new way of seeing myself, and each new pose—Relaxation Pose with eyes closed or

Downward-Facing Dog Pose or Half Moon Pose or Lunge Pose or Cobra Pose or Plank Pose—helped change my perspective on the world. Instead of always striving to achieve, I found myself content to just be, to experience the present moment without rushing to the next or looking back on what I might have missed. The asanas not only led my body into new ways of moving, they led me into new ways of being, new ways of seeing. They helped root me in the present moment. But before I could truly see, I had to be willing to bare my feet and pay attention.

JOURNAL PRACTICE: PAYING ATTENTION

➤ Sit on your mat (or chair) with your journal nearby. Review the times during the day when you judged yourself or viewed yourself in a critical light. Notice the critical voice. You don't need to respond to or argue with the voice, just listen, as painful as it may be to hear what it has to say. Pay attention to the inflections, the sound, the things that it criticizes, the way the voice tries to discourage you or undermine your efforts. When you can hear that voice clearly, open your journal and let that voice come through your pen onto the page. Is it a voice that you recognize as belonging to someone you know? A close relative? A friend? Let the voice exhaust itself. Just write until the voice has nothing left to criticize, until the voice is silent and your pen stops moving.

Now close your eyes and take ten gentle rounds of breath. Then open your eyes and write about how you feel now, in this moment, when the critical voice is silent. Can you recognize your own voice as distinct from but part of the critical voice? How can you accept that critical voice without pushing it away? How can you tap into your own voice more often and more deeply? Ask yourself why the critical voice is so critical. In writing about it, you may find a new way of understanding it and why you respond the way you do. Write for five minutes at first. See where that leads you.

▶ Are you ashamed or embarrassed by a part of your body? Use your journal to explore your feelings. What is it about your body that embarrasses you? Did you always feel this way, or is it a recent discovery? Describe the part of your body that you find embarrassing. How can you change the way you look at your body so your feelings change, too? Are you comparing yourself to someone else or to an ideal? Why do you feel the need to compare yourself to someone else? How can you learn to view yourself and your body without judgment? Use your journal to describe your body, and notice whenever you find yourself feeling ashamed or embarrassed. Then explore those feelings in more depth. Ask yourself what quality you might want to develop so you can begin to accept your body as it is, and then write about that quality. See if you can cultivate that quality in your daily life, and try to notice it in yourself and in others. What if you pay attention to this quality for a week or even a month and record your feelings about it in your journal each day?

➤ Use your journal to describe each moment, each breath. What are you feeling now? And now? A breeze against your skin? An itch on the bottom of your big toe? And what are you sensing? A tight knot in your stomach? A vague sense of unease or anxiousness? Use your body as a resource for understanding how you approach life from moment to moment. Is there a part of your body that feels tense or uncomfortable while you're sitting on your mat? What causes the tension to arise? Can you follow the tension back to a thought or image? Explore that image or that thought to understand what is causing the tension. Listen closely to your heart beating, pay attention to when it speeds up or slows down. Write as you listen, and let your pen take you from one moment to the next until you reach a point of stillness. Then put aside your journal and begin your practice, trying to stay in the moment of each pose. Afterward you can pick up your journal and write about the challenge of staying in the present—not leaping ahead in your mind to worries about the future, not sinking into regrets about the past or what you might have done. Stay in the present as it unfolds, moment to moment, and try to discern what you feel now—and now.

5: Awakening to Connections

It was a gentle feeling, not a straining to unite or join,
more like a caress, a kiss, a reminder of the limitlessness of my spirit.
—FROM MY JOURNAL

When I began my yoga practice, I was unaware of the connection between the challenges that I faced on the mat and those that I encountered in my daily life. But over time, the more I practiced and the more I reflected on that practice in my journal, the connection became clearer.

The first time I remember realizing that there was a connection, I was driving to class. I had left the house a few minutes later than usual, so I rushed to the car and sped off, thinking I had to get to class on time or I'd miss my favorite part, the introductory theme of the class that Rita shared with us in a circle before we began our asanas. I also didn't want to miss the casual banter among the students as we stretched and warmed up on our mats. That was one of the gifts of the class, hearing about the lives of the other students and sharing my life with them.

But how was I going to arrive on time if I had to stop the car before getting a quarter mile from the house because a pair of sandhill cranes were strolling across the road? I couldn't believe my eyes. I was trying to get to class, and my way was blocked by these birds! For readers who have never seen them, these tall, beautiful birds have toothpick-thin legs, dark, needle-like beaks, and elegant necks that look like supple tubes of gray silk. Their foreheads of bright scarlet feathers flash red against their tawny wing feathers and sleek, silver bodies. But I was not interested in their handsome display that morning. I sat behind the wheel of my car getting more and more impatient as the birds took their time walking across the road, pausing in front of my car to inspect the driver (who was now cursing behind the windshield). Finally, the birds made it safely onto the grassy curb. I pressed my foot to the floor and sped away, checking my watch and praying that I still had time to make it to the class before Rita began the lesson.

But it was late November. If you know Florida and its influx of residents and visitors each winter, you know late November is considered "the season" here. The roads are clogged with cars bearing license plates from Michigan, Ohio, Illinois, New York, Pennsylvania, North Carolina, Missouri, Iowa, Maine, and parts of Canada. I may have made it successfully past the sandhill cranes, but I still had to contend with traffic—traffic at the light at the end of my street, traffic on the four-lane parkway leading to the highway, traffic on the highway. Even side roads, clear most of the year, were clogged with traffic that morning, so my decision to take the local roads didn't help me escape the line of cars backed up ahead of me.

I looked at my watch. The minutes were ticking away. At this moment, I told myself, the students in class would be warming up. I glanced at my watch again a few minutes later. Now they'll be closing the door to begin, I thought. I stared at my watch, trying to keep the seconds from advancing, wishing I could stop time just long enough to make it to class before Rita shut the door. But time refused to stand still, unlike the cars, which hadn't moved in the last five minutes.

I made it to within a mile of the yoga center when the traffic halted again. It was backed up around the bend, a half mile ahead. I prayed the cars would start to flow and I might slip into the class without anyone noticing that I was late, assuming I could reach the center in the next five minutes and find a parking spot. But when the car ahead of me flashed its brake lights and came to a stop, my hopes came to a stop, too. I slumped over the wheel, shaking my head, defeated. I was not going to make it. The traffic was backed up ahead of me due to a construction crew that I could see now digging on the side of the road to repair an underground pipe. I was convinced that we'd never move again, and that I'd have to live out the remainder of my life trapped in traffic.

And then I glanced past the car ahead of me at the woods on the side of the road. It was November, and in Florida the leaves don't turn colors the way they do farther north. But these woods were filled with colors—the green of palm trees and long-needle pines and live oak, the grayish-green wisps of Spanish moss hanging from the branches, the brown leaves of sycamores, and the honey-golden sunlight suffusing the trees with that rare autumn glow, soft and gauzelike and so thick I could almost touch it. I felt my eyes open as I looked into the woods, forgetting for a moment the line of cars I was stuck in and the class I was missing. I simply let the woods and the colors and the light fill me up. It felt as if time had stopped for a moment, just long enough for me to notice the beauty surrounding me. And in that moment of recognition, I stopped wanting to be somewhere else. I stopped rushing, pushing, shoving myself out of the moment and just sat staring at the woods—the tree trunks painted with light, the leaves glimmering gold—and I realized just how lucky I was to notice such beauty, to be a part of this world.

And I had to laugh at myself for being such a fool, for being blind to this beauty and, earlier, to the beauty of the sandhill cranes crossing the road. What difference did it make if I got to the class on time, I asked myself? I was here, now, and this was the moment given to me. Not some moment waiting for me (which might never come or I might never reach). Not some moment in the past, but this moment, now. Wasn't this exactly what I was trying to learn through yoga, how to appreciate each moment of life?

So, sitting in my car, I felt as if I'd given myself my first yoga lesson. In my mind, I could see myself learning the different poses—Standing Forward Bend Pose, Lunge Pose, Plank Pose, Cobra Pose, Downward-Facing Dog Pose—and flowing from one to the other. But until that moment I hadn't connected the way we practice the flow of poses with the flow of my own life. Each challenge that we face, whether it's finding ourselves stuck in traffic or facing unexpected surgery or encountering difficulties in a relationship, is a pose of sorts. We respond to the challenge in much the same way that our bodies respond to the challenge of a difficult pose. We might complain or protest or deny that we're feeling any pain at all. But my work on the mat has taught me to notice these details, to pay attention to my inner voice, to explore the sensations my body is feeling, to understand the pose and embody it fully and move on to the next pose, letting go of the one before it.

FROM MY JOURNAL

 We do lots of twists and forward bends. We do a pranayama exercise, on our backs, resting on three blankets, our legs stretched out in front of us, breathing into our lungs in three stages—a full belly, the section above the naval, and beneath our clavicles—as if our lungs are divided into three separate compartments—and breathing into these compartments (and breathing out again) one section at a time to deepen our breath and make us more conscious of the breath's presence, its life-giving effects.

Even now, as I write, I hear my breath. And hearing it lets me slow down. I feel calmer, even as I have to prepare in thirty minutes for an afternoon writing workshop.

After mat: The flow between poses makes me aware of the connectedness of membranes, muscles, and bones. Energy and spirit rush through the blood, fill the lungs and heart with life. With each pose the stiffness melts away. By the end, when I go

into my series of standing balance poses (tree, half moon, eagle),
the stiffness is gone, leaving only pure energy, and a kind of
contentment in feeling the movement of my body, the bending
of joints, the exhalation and inhalation of air.

The journal, too, is part of this practice of noticing and awakening to connections. The act of writing helps me see my thoughts as they appear. And that visibility helps me understand them differently, on a physical level. By putting words on paper, by holding a pen in my hand and moving my hand across the page, I'm bringing thoughts into the world, luring them from the realm of the abstract to assume a physical reality, a physical connection to the world.

So, sitting in my car, stuck in traffic, I let go of my wish to make it to class on time. I let go of my fear of being embarrassed to walk in late. I let go of my desire to participate in the preclass warm-up and introduction. I let go of it all. There will always be next week, or the week after that, I thought. What have I missed, really?

By the time the traffic began moving again and I found a parking spot and entered the class, I'd only missed ten minutes. The class was just getting started because other students had been stuck in traffic, too, and, like me, were arriving late. Even after I rolled out my mat and found a place in the circle, students kept coming in, and we laughed because everyone shared the same frustrations and worries about being late to class.

That morning in our circle, before beginning our asanas, I shared the story of how I'd missed the beauty of the sandhill cranes and would have missed the beauty of the woods, too, if I hadn't stopped rushing and opened my eyes. "What am I spending all this time on the mat for," I asked the others, "if not to find inner peace? I thought I'd learned how to find it. But I guess I needed to learn the lesson again." Inner peace isn't something that comes easily to me. It's something that I seek daily and find only rarely, usually in unexpected moments

JOURNAL PRACTICE: AWAKENING TO CONNECTIONS

► Notice, as you perform your daily practice, which pose gives you the most difficulty. Is it a balancing pose? Or a back bend? Or perhaps an inversion, such as Headstand or Handstand? Without opening your journal, sit for a moment envisioning yourself moving into the pose that gives you the greatest difficulty. Close your eyes. Imagine yourself balancing in Tree Pose, if that's the one that gives you a problem. Or imagine yourself upside down in Handstand. Whatever pose it might be, let your mind draw you into it slowly, so you can see each movement that you must make in order to bring your body into that pose. Can you see what's keeping you from arriving at the pose? A fear, perhaps, of standing on one leg and falling? Or the embarrassment of standing on your head? Or the dread of taking a risk and failing? Once you've identified the issue that's keeping you from fully stepping into the pose, open your journal and begin to write about that issue. Use the process of writing about the pose to help you find a way to overcome your fear or embarrassment or dread. Write about how practicing yoga helps you connect with deeper layers of yourself. Use specific examples from your life.

> Begin to notice, as you go through your day, how you respond to difficult situations. If you're stuck in traffic, for instance, or waiting on line at the grocery store, do you find yourself growing impatient, frustrated, angry that you're not moving faster? Or, say, you meet a friend, and the conversation takes an unexpected turn, and you're suddenly upset, facing a critic instead of an admirer, hearing words that are painful instead of uplifting. How do you stay in the moment without losing your temper or patience? How is encountering frustration or anger in your life mirrored when you practice a difficult asana? The next time you find yourself in a difficult pose on the mat, think of how the emotion that it evokes might resemble a similar emotion in a difficult situation off the mat, and then write about how the two emotions resemble each other and how the two situations evoke similar responses.

6: Trusting the Process

Think about how each moment has the potential
of leading you to the place where you need to be.
—FROM MY JOURNAL

....

One of the most difficult things to learn in life is trust—trust in yourself and in others, trust in the process of moving from pose to pose, trust that you'll find what you need in each moment. If the practice of yoga has taught me anything, it's that learning to trust isn't just a possibility; it's a necessity if you want to reach your full potential.

The first time I understood this on an emotional and physical level, not just an intellectual one, was when I was learning to do Camel Pose, which requires that you trust in your ability to reach backward into the unknown in an intense back bend. Unless you have confidence in yourself, in your body's ability to attain the pose, and in the invisible force supporting you, you'll never lean back far enough to reach your heels.

The process of preparing for this pose and then actually

....

attempting it helped me discover how trust is part of any pose. It's as essential as my legs and feet, which serve as foundation of Camel Pose, and my lower spine, which allows me to extend upward into my upper back and shoulders and downward into my hips and thighs. It's as essential as my arms, which reach back into the emptiness, and my hands, which grasp my heels.

Trust in the universal energy flowing through all of life, trust that I'll be given what I need in the moment, is what allows me to lean backward into that emptiness. Whether I reach my heels is unimportant; it's the process of reaching for my heels, the willingness to strive for something beyond my reach, that links me to that flow of energy, helps me feel it flowing through me. Trust is what gives me the strength to close my eyes and see what I can't see: a path to a new way of understanding myself and my body that only moments before had been hidden from view. And it's trust that compels me to follow that path without knowing where it will lead, in the belief that I will discover a new perspective and find a new vantage point from which to view life. Looking back now, I think that all along, from the moment I decided to remove my shoes and socks and step onto the mat, the process of learning and exploring poses has been about learning to have faith in myself and others and learning, too, to trust in the universal energy that is larger than us all.

Camel Pose, for those who may not know it, is a challenging— some might even say intense—back bend. When I kneel on the mat, toes tucked under, I root my knees and toes into the earth as I reach for the sky, lifting my head and shoulders, and then I bring my arms down behind me and lower my hands to reach for my heels, leaning farther back into the pose. As I reach for my heels, that ultimate moment of surrender, I can't see my hands or my feet, and it feels as if I'm reaching into a void. In order to reach my heels, I have to trust, as I lean farther and farther backward, pushing past doubts and discomfort, that my feet are there and my hands are where they're supposed to be, and if I just keep leaning, keep breathing deeply, I'll find my heels. I have to believe that I'll find what I need. Without trust, I couldn't reach the full expression of this pose.

Our practice of Camel Pose each week first made me aware of trust as a crucial element in each pose. But it was our exploration of a new pose that deepened my understanding of the nature of trust. Shortly after we'd explored Camel Pose, Rita introduced us to Revolved Extended Side-Angle Pose, which is a lunge of sorts, but with a twist added to make it more interesting.

In Lunge Pose, you extend one leg straight behind you, while the other leg is bent so the knee is positioned directly above the ankle. Your hips are level, at the same height as your forward knee, and you lean forward over your bent knee and reach for the floor with the fingertips of both hands. But in Revolved Extended Side-Angle Pose, if your left knee is placed in front, then you twist to the left, reaching with your right hand across the top of your left thigh so your elbow is positioned just beyond your leg. Then you bend your elbow and bring your hands together in Prayer Position and lean back slightly.

That's the description of the physical pose, but it doesn't describe how the pose helps alter my perception of where I am and what I can do in the world, or how my breath comes faster the deeper I lean into the pose, or how I struggle to find my balance, or how I need to pull back from a twist so I don't keel over. Each pose asks for a constant adjustment of positions and a constant refinement of awareness. Nor does the physical description hint at the emotional challenges that I face getting into the position and holding the pose. It's that effort of leaning back, even slightly, that requires me to have faith in the force of the universe, an invisible source of energy that supports us all, so I can bend backward into a fuller expression of the pose.

Every part of the pose requires trust, from the moment I step into the lunge—before I even begin to twist—to the moment I press my hands together in front of my heart and lean backward slightly into the unknown. The lunge itself requires poise and balance. But I need to trust myself to be able to hold my balance, especially in the most extreme point of the pose. Each of these poses—Camel Pose, Lunge Pose, Revolved Extended Side-Angle Pose—helped me change the way I viewed the poses and understand that confidence is an essential component of every pose.

From My Journal

I'm thinking as I step onto the mat about freedom. How it can come from the very restraints that one's body can impose. Yet how in a particular pose, with a specific form, you can find freedom. Freedom to think and feel in different ways before and after experiencing the restraints. And also: not to view all restraints as negative, all impasses as fruitless encounters.

Can you view such obstacles as harbingers of grace, moments that open us to the possibilities hidden in ourselves, drawing out strength and courage that we weren't aware of before meeting the restraint?

Even before you step on the mat, you need confidence if you expect to experience the fullness of the universe and the fullness of your own potential. You are always one hundred percent yourself in each pose, whether you find your way into its fullness or simply reach toward it. That moment of reaching—that is the full expression of your potential in that moment. Each pose offers us the possibility to challenge our notions of ourselves, our assumptions about life and our place in the world, and gives us a way to learn something new about our untapped possibilities.

Even Relaxation Pose, in which you lie motionless on your back, legs slightly parted, hands and feet slightly splayed, eyes closed, can lead to new insights. The simple act of lying on your back in a room full of strangers and closing your eyes requires trust, doesn't it? Who is the woman beside you, the man at the front of the room? Who is the teacher, and can I trust him to lead us through the poses safely? Will the teacher allow me to be myself, so I can relax and expand? Or will the teacher's approach lead me to want to hide behind a mask and contract? On some days, trust is impossible. It's a wisp of fog, a thread of mist carried away by the wind. I feel abandoned, wary of everything. On days when I don't know where to find trust, it's hard to have confidence in myself. Trust requires a leap of faith.

When you walk into a yoga class for the first time, not knowing anyone, not knowing what to do, you have to trust in whatever inspired you to take that first step, and then you have to take the next step and the next, trusting in the process of discovery. This abiding confidence in the process of life unfolding demands a certain amount of faith in yourself. You need to be willing to take risks, to make mistakes, to fail. Trusting the process gives you the ability to overcome setbacks and obstacles and, rather than despair, take joy in discovering the next step and the next.

But if you're like me, faith and confidence don't come easily. It can be a struggle to just lie on your mat, close your eyes, and let go of anxieties. Just being in the moment—listening to your breath, feeling your chest rising up and down, softening your skin so you can feel the breath from your nostrils brush across your lips—requires trust. It can take years until you trust yourself enough to simply lie still, your thoughts quiet, your mind relaxed, and listen to the stillness without needing to go anywhere else. Working through a variety of poses, even the most basic, teaches you how to trust yourself. How? By helping you learn to listen to your body. Listen: Does your abdomen or chest feel tense? Listen: Do your neck or shoulders feel strained? Listen: Do your hips or lower back feel relaxed? These sensations reveal the state of your body, but they also express the state of your mind and your heart.

When I first stepped onto the mat, I wasn't even aware that my body was trying to tell me something. I typically sat for hours every day typing at my desk, my neck and back aching, ignoring the pain so I could finish my work. Then I'd run until I could barely breathe, my thighs and calves burning as if the muscles, tendons, and joints were ablaze. I'd ignore the pain, thinking that pain was a sign of a good workout. A good workout was one that allowed me to conquer pain, to run through it, as we used to say. No pain, no gain. That was our high school coach's favorite expression, and he said it often. It wasn't until my body broke under the stress of pain that I began to question the merits of such training methods.

It was as a junior in high school that I developed Achilles tendinitis and, essentially, ruined my legs and any chance that I might have had of running competitively. With that kind of injury, I was lucky I hadn't crippled myself for life. Cortisone injections didn't help. Hot compresses didn't help. Ultrasound treatments didn't help. Ice didn't help. For weeks I stayed off my feet as much as possible. That's hard when you're used to running ten to fifteen miles a day. I put heel inserts in my shoes. I walked gingerly, trying to keep the weight off my toes. I soaked my ankles every night, then iced the Achilles tendons. Nothing helped—except rest.

What had I learned from my injury? Not until I began practicing yoga did I view the experience in terms of trust. I had been taught not to trust my body but rather to ignore its signals of pain and distress. In the process of trusting my coach and my friends (who were all pushing themselves as hard as I was), I had learned to disregard myself. If I heard a voice of protest or complaint, I quickly silenced it. If I heard a voice of doubt, I ignored it. I didn't pay attention to that inner voice until the intense pain in my ankles forced me to recognize it. Instead of helping me reach my full potential, my coach and fellow runners had helped me curtail it. And I realized that if I kept listening to other people and ignoring my own voice, I'd destroy my potential and any chance of reaching it.

Unlike my coach's philosophy of no pain, no gain, which taught me to ignore my body, Jaye's philosophy of no pain, no pain (which he discovered in Judith Hanson Lasater's *Living Your Yoga*) is a gentle reminder that we must always listen to our bodies and trust ourselves to know when to back away from a pose that's too intense or a position that's too challenging. We can't place our faith in others to tell us when to stop. We need to know ourselves and trust that we can decide by listening closely and understanding that pain is a serious warning. Your body is trying to send you a message. *Listen.*

The ongoing conversation with your body is a crucial element in the process of learning to trust yourself. You start with your body and accept where it is when you step on the mat. Beginning with Cat Tilt and Dog Tilt, you listen to your knees and hips. You listen to the vertebrae in your spine and neck. You move, and with each movement you listen to what your body is telling you, and you make adjustments in your pose to suit your body's needs in that moment. In Mountain Pose, you raise your arms over your head and listen to your shoulders. And then in Standing Forward Bend, you bow forward and listen to your lower back, your hamstrings, your ankles. What do you hear? Do you need to ease off a little? Or can you move more deeply into the pose? Intensity is different than pain. What is your body telling you to do? Listen. Trust the process.

With that trust, you'll notice how much more closely you pay attention to your practice and your feelings about it. And just as you learn to trust your body on the mat, you learn to trust it when you step off the mat, too. Long after you leave your yoga class and drive to work or back home, you keep listening. Did I do too much, push too hard? Did I mistake pain for intensity? Did I go far enough?

And off the mat, you listen to your body in each situation as it arises during the day—an argument with a teenage daughter, a tense discussion about finances with a spouse, a silent vigil with a dying parent. You begin to notice how your body feels when your boss yells at you or your sister fails to call or you miss the last showing of a movie that you've wanted to see for months. And as you listen to your body in these situations, just as you listen to it on the mat, you begin to see how your responses help you or hinder you from living life to its fullest.

You begin to recognize certain behavior as nonproductive, even destructive, contracting the world around you, and you notice other patterns of behavior as helpful, productive, bringing you in closer touch with yourself and expanding your world. The more we trust ourselves, the more the world will respond with greater opportunities to expand and grow.

FROM MY JOURNAL

The world makes a place for each of us when we enter the world, it opens to welcome us. Yet sometimes we are blind to the space that is our space and feel there is no space—no place—for us; we feel tight and constricted, searching for that place.

The key is in opening your heart, giving your heart to whatever arouses your interest, whatever sparks your passion. Once you open to create the space for your heart, you can relax and sink into that space.

Journal Practice: Trusting the Process

» With your journal open in your lap, write down the word *trust* in the middle of a blank page. Then draw a vertical line beneath it that extends to the bottom of the page. On one side, write the word *Yes;* on the other side of the line, write *No.* Then list the things or people or experiences that you trust in your life on the *Yes* side, and list the things you don't trust on the *No* side. Things you might trust: a best friend, the taste of an orange popsicle on a hot night, the wind blowing off the sea. Things you might not trust: a teacher, knives, an exspouse, rain or snow or ice on pavements, potholes. A week later you might want to review the list to see what, if anything, has changed and then write about the change.

» Continue using your journal to explore trust in your life. Write about a time when you found your faith in a person rewarded. Then write about a time when you found yourself hurt because of a betrayal of trust. What was different in each situation? What led to the positive feelings and what led to the negative feelings? How did you perceive trust before each experience and then afterward? And how did the experience change you?

▸ How do you develop trust? On the mat, you can develop trust in incremental stages as you explore a certain pose. Each step fosters greater confidence, as you perform more and more challenging tasks, and with it comes the poise to remain in the pose, even when it becomes difficult.

On your mat, pick an asana that is difficult for you, a balancing pose, for instance, or a back bend, and work your way into it slowly. Notice when you can trust your body and when you begin to lose confidence in it. What allows you to trust your body to do the pose? How can you take the trust that you develop on the mat and transfer it to your life, so you can feel more confident in more and more varied situations? Write about your feelings of trust and about the situations that encourage those feelings to contract or expand.

7: Just Sitting

By the end of the session I found my thoughts meandering
rather than rushing. I could accept them, let them go,
accept one more, let it go. Just watching. No judgment.
—FROM MY JOURNAL

When was the last time you simply sat still without needing to go anywhere and closed your eyes, welcoming each thought or sensation as it appeared, letting it go, and welcoming the next? Until I began practicing yoga, I sat at a desk writing or in a chair reading, but I never simply sat. Sitting involves becoming aware, and, for the most part, whenever I sat down to write or to read, I wanted to lose myself in other worlds, either those of my own creation or those that others had created. In fact, looking back, I would say that sitting in that way helped me run away from myself.

But sitting in yoga, in Easy Pose, for instance, where you cross your legs at the ankles and extend your spine straight up and bring your head and neck into alignment with your shoulders and rest your hands loosely, palms up or palms down, on your knees—that kind of sitting encourages you to pay attention to yourself and your relationship to the world. It's not easy at first. At least it wasn't easy for me, which was puzzling because, after all, how difficult can it be to sit? But in time I discovered that sitting isn't just sitting.

When I first started taking classes at the Garden of the Heart Yoga Center, the first thing I noticed when Vesna asked us to sit during class was that I had no distractions to take me away from myself—no book, no journal, no pen, no computer, no phone. There was just the mat, my body, and me. Suddenly I was aware of muscles and joints that I had forgotten all about. After a few minutes of "just" sitting, I could feel my hip bones pressing into the mat, my buttocks sinking into the floor, and the pressure of one leg against the other. It wasn't painful, but after a few minutes it no longer felt comfortable.

Everyone else looked so relaxed, and Vesna looked so tranquil and calm, the expression on her face like the reflection of a still pool. But me? I felt pain in my hips and tension in my abdominal muscles. It took a lot of effort to sit erect for so long and not let the physical sensations of pain or discomfort disturb me. And it took greater restraint not to move out of the pose, to remain seated, to explore the position and what my body was trying to tell me, not with words but with sensations.

That first sitting didn't last long—a few minutes, perhaps, five at most. But time seemed to expand. My mind magnified the pain until it seemed that everything hurt, even my little toe as it pressed into the mat to help me keep my balance. Was the pain real or was I imagining it? Would the pose hurt me or help me? Should I have uncrossed my legs to come out of the pose sooner, despite what others were doing? These questions were the beginning of my yoga practice, the door into yoga for me. This one pose, just sitting, taught me that I could be with myself and not run from things I might find disturbing, things that I might not want to face.

Just as I had to learn to explore the discomfort of a certain pose and discover that I could sit with the discomfort, so did I have to learn how to explore certain aspects of my life—my personality, my relationships with members of my family and with friends, the way I often ran from a challenge rather than standing up to it—and to sit with these realizations without allowing them to frighten me away.

In time, over the course of a year or two, I noticed that I began to sit differently, not just in my yoga practice but in my daily work. On the mat, as various asanas like Boat Pose and Plank Pose helped strengthen my abdominal muscles, I found myself able to sit with less discomfort. I no longer felt my stomach muscles clench after a few minutes. I could sit erect, spine tall, chin balanced above my chest, and feel relaxed, as if I was viewing my own reflection in a still pond, tranquil and serene.

Instead of noticing aches and pains or discomfort, I noticed the way my breath flowed through my nose, the slight current of air against my upper lip. I noticed how my bones fit into one another like a snug jigsaw puzzle, balanced, at ease. And I noticed how my muscles were relaxed, held to the bone but with grace and lightness, no longer clenched and tight. I was paying attention to the way my body felt in the moment, and because I was no longer tense, I could focus on my thoughts as they arose, could stay with a thought as long as I needed to, and then could let go and allow another thought to appear. If no thoughts arose, I simply sat and enjoyed that space. After all, thinking is not the point of sitting. As the minutes passed, the need to distance myself from my self disappeared. I no longer sought distractions; instead, I began to look for ways to go deeper.

This shift in perspective, this change in attitude, affected how I read books and wrote stories and related to friends and family. It came as a result of hours of sitting and then more hours of asking myself what I'd experienced on the mat and noting down my responses and additional questions in my journal. Why do I run from challenges? Is that indeed true, or do I assume it's true because someone once told me that? Why do I have trouble talking to my father? Why do I feel close to my brother but can't tell him? Why am I angry so much of the time, while smiling to conceal the anger?

As each question arose, as painful as it was to consider, I sat with it. I wrote the question down on paper. I let it swirl around in my mind. I didn't run. I didn't get up from my chair or mat and leave the room. I didn't put down my pen and close my journal. I sat and listened and tried to pay attention to what my body— and my heart—was telling me. I learned how to take a breath if I found myself tensing up. I learned to "listen" to the muscles in the pit of my stomach and noticed that they clenched tighter and tighter the more troubling the question I asked myself.

But I continued to sit, because sitting on the mat had taught me how to sit with discomfort until I could look at a question impartially, from a neutral perspective, as if it were a question that I was asking about someone else, not myself.

FROM MY JOURNAL

Overflowing w/anger after yesterday's session—or maybe w/ memories of anger—over my mother's death 30 years ago. How unfair it seemed to lose her when she was so young—only fifty-one—and how powerless it made me feel when neither medicine nor prayers could save her.

Why this anger . . . and why now? And why did the notion of letting go of anger rekindle this intense feeling of anger, as if her death had occurred only yesterday? If I was supposed to learn to let go, to accept life as it unfolded, why was letting go impossible? No matter how hard I tried to let go, to rid myself of this anger, it clung to me—as if my hands were made of velcro or sticky glue. Why?

Today I'm not angry, just stunned by the emotions that surfaced yesterday. Where did they come from? I thought—truly believed—that I'd moved past anger into a different zone—where I accepted death as part of life. But maybe I still view her death—all deaths—as unjust? As if the game of life were rigged unfairly against us.

I don't know what kind of practice will unfold today. If I try to make more room, more spaciousness, will that merely open myself up to more anger—more disappointment—more frustration? Will it only open the floodgates of past failures, and the emotions attendant on them, rather than make space for new ways of seeing the world?

I began to open up in the pose. And, as I opened up, the answers began to emerge. Why did I run from challenges? It wasn't the challenge itself that I ran from, it was the criticism that I had come to expect from myself or others that made me shy about taking on challenges. What was the source of the criticism? Was it merely a figment of my imagination, an excuse that I made up to mask my own cowardice? Or was it real?

The answer to that question is linked, perhaps not surprisingly, to my relationship with my father, a man I loved dearly but who was always reticent about talking about himself or his life. (He died while I was working on this book.) In all the years that I knew him, he rarely revealed his feelings about anything—his job, his family, his youth, his attitudes toward God and religion, nothing. I think I interpreted his silence as rejection. I assumed I'd done something wrong (or not the way he'd have done it) for him not to offer some kind word of reassurance, some faint praise. And, to make matters worse, whenever he did say something—offer advice, make a suggestion—he offered it in the form of criticism, or perhaps that's just the way I heard it: *You shouldn't have done that* or *It would have been better if you'd tried it this way* or *How can you think like that?* The result of his silence and his criticism was to make me wary of getting too close, of sharing too much.

Ironically, my father's silence led to my own silence and ultimately to my discovery of the page (and the miracle of pen and paper) as a safe place to express myself, a place where his criticism couldn't reach me. Yet there are days when, even though he's gone, I still hear his critical voice in my head. It's the voice that I run from, not the challenges themselves. I need space from that voice, and freedom from criticism, if I'm ever going to escape from the fear and doubt that such criticism can generate, if I'm ever going to hear my own voice without hearing it filtered through my father's voice. Sitting helped me discover this, and keeping a journal helped me clarify and then refine these thoughts.

Why am I so close to my brother yet unable to tell him how much I love him? That's another question that sitting helped me answer. The last time I told anyone in our family that I loved them, they died, and I'm afraid of it happening again. Sounds silly, doesn't it? How can I believe my words have the power to bring death or misfortune to someone I love? Yet that's how I felt when I lost my mother to cancer. I was twenty-two, she was fifty-one, and my brother was eighteen. I think we were afraid we had loved her too much, that our loving her had somehow brought on her illness and ultimate death. I didn't want it to happen again, not with my brother or my wife or anyone. So I stopped saying, "I love you."

Sitting and writing in my journal week after week helped me

see this and understand how the grief and suffering of a twenty-two-year-old distorted reality and altered it to conform to my deepest fears. Those fears have shaped my life for years—but no longer. I can sit now, my journal open in my lap, my pen poised above the page, and look at my grief and the loss of my mother and understand that love played no part in her death; if anything, it helped ease her pain, even if it caused us greater pain to lose her. Words—the words that I set down in my journal, as well as the words that I say or keep to myself—have a lot of power. I'm aware that I can hurt another person's feelings with words, even change their view of reality. But words don't have the power to bring about death any more than love does. Words can separate or they can bring people closer. Writing years later in my journal about my family and my relationship with my father helped me understand this.

I have yet to summon the courage to tell my brother how much I love him. Fear lingers—superstitious fear, but fear nonetheless. But soon I hope we'll sit down and I'll look at him across the table in his dining room or at one of our favorite New Jersey diners and see in his face a reflection of our mother's love and our father's determination, and I'll tell him how much he means to me without fearing that I'll lose him the moment I utter the words.

And the anger that I harbor in my heart but keep hidden? What about that? It's not the kind of anger that flares up quickly and dies away again. It's a slow burn, a steady, simmering anger that began the night my mother died and God kept silent, and no reason was offered, no explanation given, for why such a kind-hearted woman should be taken from life so young or why she needed to suffer so greatly (from colon cancer that spread to her liver) over the last six months of her life.

I was angry at the doctors for not saving her, angry at my father for not doing something, for not saying something to us earlier. (He kept it a secret between him and the doctor until the illness progressed to the point where the truth could no longer be hidden.) Most of all, I was angry at God for establishing a world where you had to let go of the people you loved the most. And the anger fed on itself through the year of mourning, and afterward it never really burned out, just kept simmering.

It wasn't until I started sitting on my yoga mat that I began to understand the depth of my rage and the intensity of my disappointment in prayer and in God. Why did Mom have to suffer? Why did life have to change? For years I struggled with these questions. But as I sat, I began to understand. Just as different poses prove challenging and sometimes painful, life is sometimes challenging and painful. Just as our poses change as we go from one asana to the next, so too do our lives change moment to moment. It is the nature of life to change. Change, I began to see, is the essence of life. We can no more keep life from transforming than we can hold back the tide from rising on the shore.

There is still a remnant of anger in my heart, a need to protest what seemed—and still seems—like an injustice. But now it's an anger that includes and has been softened by the understanding that my mother wasn't singled out by God for suffering. Every day innocent people suffer, some far worse than she did—victims of earthquakes, floods, hurricanes, illness, disease. It is the nature of life, not something to reject (although you can try to alleviate suffering). It's rather something to accept as part of life's unfolding. Such acceptance can lead to a deeper understanding of what it means to be alive.

Now, each time I sit on my mat, I remind myself that I'm not just sitting. I am connecting to a source of energy deep in my heart and, at the same time, connecting to a larger source of energy, a life force that is at the core of the universe. Touching that source of energy helps me feel a greater awareness of the blood pulsing through my veins, the breath filling my lungs, the life that we all share. And it's that source of energy that enables me to accept the world and life not as I might want it to be but as it is.

FROM MY JOURNAL

 Yesterday I tried to explain the attractiveness of yoga to friends. I told them how it feels less like a workout, more like a search for balance, and how the flow of poses make my body feel like a living Cat's Cradle. And how the lessons you learn on the mat about patience and faith and self-confidence can be transforming off the mat as well.

New poses challenge not just your body—and your expectations of what your body can do—but your mind. Perhaps new

forms, new poses, I suggest, help enlarge your way of thinking
about yourself and the world, and actually stimulate new brain
cells. It's important at a certain age to keep your mind and body
limber, to push the edges a bit . . . and make new discoveries.

Journal Practice: Just Sitting

» Listen to your body as you sit on your mat. Cross your legs,
relax your arms, let your tongue loosen, and then close your
eyes (or keep them open if you prefer). Just sit. Notice what
you feel—a twinge in a muscle, an ache in your neck, a
numb tingling along your calf—without judging or evalu-
ating it. With your eyes still closed, move gradually from
what you feel to what you think. Notice the thoughts that
float through your mind, the images that come up out of the
darkness and then fade, replaced by others. Let your mind
empty itself of images, and focus only on your breath—in
and out, in and out. Spend at least five minutes sitting. At
the end of five minutes, open your journal and describe the
sensations that were most difficult for you to accept and
those that put you at ease. How did you sit through the
difficult sensations? What was it like to come up against an
unexpected difficulty and then move through it? What was
it like to feel at ease while sitting?

» Sitting on your mat with your notebook open in your lap,
begin writing about a person who you find difficult to be

with. Imagine a situation in which you and this person meet. Describe what the situation looks like from your perspective, and then describe what the situation looks like from the other person's perspective. What does he or she see, and how does it differ from what you see? How long can you "sit" with this person? Write about the difference between learning to sit through a difficult pose and learning to sit with a difficult person. And then write about how the two experiences are similar or different.

» Sitting can serve as a catalyst for change. Isn't that ironic? From a motionless position, we are catapulted into movement. Make a list of the things in your life that seem static, unchanging, that are weighing you down. Sit with them. Let yourself move into them slowly and explore them. Try to understand what it is about these things that feels so heavy. Explain in your journal what makes these things obstacles in your life. Can you, through sitting, come to see a way to lighten these things, a way to move past them? Write about change—why you think it can happen, why you think it can't—and how you would like to see your life transform.

» How is seeking perfection different from seeking contentment? Whether you're seeking perfection in your poses or in your life, it can create enormous stress for yourself and those around you. But the moment you stop seeking perfection and instead seek contentment, then the question changes. And to answer that question, you have to ask another: What do I want? And another: What do I need? Spend ten minutes exploring the difference between these questions in your journal.

8: Finding Your Balance

It's like a game of hide-and-seek that you play with yourself
as you search for your balance on and off the mat.
—FROM MY JOURNAL

As I've progressed from one class to the next, I've come to understand how the practice of yoga—the time that I set aside to explore various poses, the days in class, the ongoing ritual of keeping a journal—helps me find my balance in life. So now, when I stand on one leg trying to balance in Tree Pose, I understand that I'm not simply trying to balance in that moment. I'm trying to develop the skills to balance in every moment of life. By balance, I mean finding the center in a dance of opposites: effort/ease, attachment/aversion, push/pull. The balance point is shifting constantly, always in motion. It is not solid or static. There is nowhere, really, to get to, because we are always moving, always arriving, if only slightly, imperceptibly, always searching for that balance point, even in Relaxation Pose. So finding my balance involves noticing where I am and how I need to adjust my stance in life as in asanas on the mat.

Tree Pose is the earliest balance pose that I learned. I never imagined then, when I was new to yoga, that the way I struggled with my balance when I lifted one leg off the mat and pressed the sole of my foot into my inner thigh and raised my arms above my head would lead to my understanding of maintaining the balance in my life. Then it was merely a pose to learn, like Downward-Facing Dog Pose or Extended Triangle Pose, and struggle to explore.

And, believe me, I struggled in the beginning. The moment I lifted one foot off the mat, I started to wobble. The standing leg started shaking, and I could barely lift the other leg off the mat for a few seconds before I had to lower it, unable to find my center of gravity, that line of energy that would keep me balanced. Instead of raising my leg and planting my foot on the inside of my thigh, I kept the ball of my foot on the ground, lifting only the heel, and I drew the heel against the ankle of the standing leg, turning out my knee so I could find balance more easily. And it worked. By keeping just the toes of one foot on the floor for support, I could balance for the length of time the rest of the class held the traditional pose. It was a small step forward, but it was a step. Each time Vesna led us into Tree Pose over the course of those early sessions, I began to gain more confidence and the strength to move my toes off the floor and the heel of my foot higher than the ankle on my standing leg. Inch by inch, I raised my heel from my calf to just above the calf, then to just above the knee. Each upward movement was a challenge and, once achieved, a grand accomplishment.

In the class, I had learned not to measure my performance against the performance of the other students. In fact, I had to learn to stop seeing the pose itself as a performance. It was instead an inner exploration of how I felt in the pose and how my life was (or was not) in balance. In time, the pose showed me not only how to balance but how to recognize when things were in balance and when they were not. It was extraordinary, really. How can standing on one foot with your arms over your head do this? But it can and it does, if you pay close attention to the changes within your body and learn to see beyond your own body.

FROM MY JOURNAL

 It's the first day of summer, and the heat is thick and heavy. Florida heat. But it feels good, loosens tense muscles, seeps into bones, releases energy. Off a week from classes, I feel a stronger desire to practice today than three days ago. I'm finding that I need yoga to stretch and restore my body's balance. Without yoga, my body constricts, my muscles tighten, and my mind closes in on itself. With yoga, my body feels light and full, restored to balance and energy. I can breathe easily, without strain. I sit cross-legged on my mat. The sun beats down on the patio beyond the shaded area where I spread my mat. Time to begin.

After mat: I'm starting to notice how slight adjustments bring

me into greater balance. Yet, without warning, I can lose my

balance, flailing arms and legs before toppling to the mat.

Years later, still struggling with balance in Tree Pose, I ask myself in the pages of my journal why I'm having such trouble with balance or with the simple act of keeping my foot pressed against my inner thigh. These questions lead me to consider issues of balance that I encounter every day in my life in ways that I'm not always aware of or, if truth be told, issues that perhaps I prefer to ignore.

For instance, even though I'm in my mid-fifties, I can still remember feeling like a teenager whenever I had a conversation with my father. No matter whether he called or I called, he always prefaced his comments with the same question: "What's new?" Now, that would seem to be an innocuous question, almost meaningless, to most people. But it carried such weight for me, such a history, that I couldn't hear it without stuttering and fumbling for an answer and feeling like a fool for not having a better one. I'm sure my father didn't intend to upset me by asking the question, but the question, and perhaps the tone that I heard in his voice when he posed it, along with my uncertainty about how to respond in order to please him, inevitably upset my balance. Every time I heard the question, I felt like my father was judging me. When he asked "What's new?" I cringed at the critical voice whispering in my ear: What have you accomplished today that's worthwhile? That's not what my father said, but it's what I heard. What's new that's made you a lot of money? What have you done to become a success? Why aren't you famous yet? To say that this question threw our relationship out of balance is an understatement. Each time we talked and my father began the conversation with this question, it was as if a gale-force wind ripped through the phone and threatened to blow me out to sea, and I always felt as if, once cast adrift, I wouldn't be able to find my way back.

It was Tree Pose—and my thoughts about the pose and the challenge of finding my balance—that helped me recognize how my father's question was throwing me off balance. The pose helped me recognize that our relationship was a pose and that the pose of our relationship could assume the balance of a sturdy tree or a wobbly and frail sapling. This was a revelation to me. It meant our relationship wasn't stagnant, didn't have to be frozen. As long as he was alive, we could each work on our pose. We could each search for ways to restore balance to the relationship. And even though he's gone now, I can still try to understand how I might have heard my father's question differently and interpret it in a way that no longer throws off my balance.

FROM MY JOURNAL

A tropical storm is forming somewhere in the Atlantic. The forecast is for it to reach Florida later this week. And a second tropical storm is gaining strength further away. The heat is rising into the 90s every afternoon, the air so heavy and thick that you'd think you'd wrapped a wet towel over your head in a steambath. And the sun—the sun is ever brighter and brighter—so intense it hurts to look outside without sunglasses to protect your eyes.

How do you welcome these "obstacles" into your life? How do you meet these challenges to your comfort? If something— heat or sunlight—feels oppressive, how do you begin to see it as part of life's wonder, rather than as simply one more thing to complain about?

The sunlight—shining so brightly that it blinds you. The heat—baking the earth to nearly scorching. As if the world, the universe, is out of balance.

So . . . standing on one leg, eyes closed, you try to find your balance . . . and restore a little of the earth's balance? Isn't that too simple? And is it even true?

All I can do, it seems, is close my eyes to shut out the sunlight and try to ignore the setting.

What do I find inside myself that lets me accept these things as part of life? How do you accept life as it is—without trying to make it into something else—cooler or shadier?

This notion of a relationship as a balance pose has changed the way I look at life. Life itself is a balance pose. Some days it's in balance, but some days we're thrown off by an unexpected deadline, a request for help, a forgotten lunch date. These things can throw off our balance as easily as two simple words framed as an innocent question. How do we maintain equanimity in the face of such daily challenges? How do we learn to accept the challenges as challenges instead of trying to combat them or deny them or run from them?

If you look closely at a tree and at Tree Pose, I think you'll find the answer. A tree, if you notice closely, *moves*. It is rooted to the ground, but it is flexible; its trunk can sway in the wind, its leaves and branches can tremble in the air. It is, in fact, a study in motion, responding to the changes in the weather or seasons. It is always changing, even if we can't always see the changes until after they occur.

In hardwoods, for instance, you can see buds emerge each spring, opening in the warm sunlight of April and May from tiny shells into leafy canopies, and you can watch the leaves unfold and grow and turn color from pale lime to a deep shade of green. Over the long, hot summer months, the leaves collect the dust and dirt of the atmosphere, and with the arrival of the cooler air of autumn they turn color and drop away. Standing naked in the snow, the tree appears motionless all winter, even though its sap is still flowing, just at a slower rate than earlier in the year.

Or look at a palm tree in a storm, how the fronds whip the air, how the trunk bends and twists but doesn't break because of its flexibility. Its roots hold the tree firm as its leaves twirl and spin and reach for the sky.

Flexibility and change: these are two aspects of trees that deepen my understanding of Tree Pose and help me apply what I discover in the pose to my life. It's taken years to be able to articulate this notion. Now I see not only my relationship with my father but my relationships with my wife and daughter as poses, too. Sometimes they're more challenging poses, sometimes easier poses, but poses nonetheless, always changing. And I'm always seeking a way to be more flexible and not as rigid in the pose, to compromise if necessary, or bend when the pose pulls me more strongly in one direction than another.

The process of keeping a journal helps me understand how I might enter a pose out of alignment and how I might regain my balance. It helps me see the pose in three dimensions rather than in only one. In this sense, the journal serves as another prop to help me go deeper into a pose, just as a block placed between my shoulder blades in Relaxation Pose might help open my chest more fully, or a folded blanket under my buttocks might help me sit straighter on the mat in Easy Pose.

My journal is also like a mirror—another prop—reflecting back to me the way I appear (to myself) in a particular pose, whether it's a pose on the mat or a relationship in my life. It lets me look at the pose with care, without hurrying, and break it down into its fundamental components. In the pages of my journal, I can examine each component of the pose and try to understand how the pieces fit together or why they fell out of balance. And thanks to the time that I spend writing in my journal, I can sometimes find a way to regain my balance if I look at the pose and think about the components long enough.

Keeping a journal helps me internalize the pose, so I can feel it inside me. Writing about the pose helps me feel through memory the way my body responds to the pose. I can feel my bones unfold again. I can feel my muscles tighten and contract. I can feel the nerves tingle with the sensation of fully embodying the pose. It's the ability to recognize when a pose is in balance and when it's not that is the first step to finding balance on the mat and in my life. Tree Pose was just the beginning. It led to the next pose and the next, just like the pages of my journal lead me from one pose to another, in an ever-changing, ever-bending dance of balance.

JOURNAL PRACTICE: FINDING YOUR BALANCE

▶ Your journal can help you find balance when you use its pages to reflect on what happens to you on the mat. If you're finding a particular pose troubling or difficult, for instance, you might ask yourself why it is such a challenge. If you're gaining insights or bits of knowledge from your asana practice, note them down on the pages of your journal. And likewise, if you're stumped, or if you've reached a crossroads, describe how you feel stuck or what two roads are crossing. Which one do you want to take? Maybe you feel like plunging into the woods and carving a new road. By paying close attention to what you write in its pages, you may be able to hear your journal responding to your words. You may not hear actual words, but you may detect the faintest of vibrations pulling you in a certain direction or discover the vaguest outline of a path to follow that will help you regain your balance.

Sit in a comfortable position on your mat or in a chair, with your journal open in your lap, and take a few moments to breathe deeply. Relax your shoulders, let the tension in your stomach melt away, and turn inward. Write about a path that you wanted to take but avoided or missed. Write about losing your balance and finding it again. Did a pose reveal something new to you about balance? Describe what you discovered and how your discovery helped you find your balance again. Write about that intimation, the feeling beneath the words, and where it might lead you.

▷ To find your balance, you must lose your balance. Start this exercise in what seems like the most stable pose of all: Table Pose. Notice how you set your foundation firmly by coming onto all fours and pressing your knees and the palms of your hands and fingertips into the mat. Then, slowly, shift your balance by lifting your left arm in front of you and, at the same time, raise your right leg behind you into Balancing Cat Pose. What happens to your balance as you bring down your arm and leg and lift the opposite arm and leg? After switching from one side to the other two or three more times, return to Table Pose to restore your stability, and then lift your left arm in front of you and your left leg behind you in a variation of Balancing Cat Pose. Notice how this pose requires an even greater effort to maintain your balance. Try the same pose on the opposite side. When you're done, move into Child's Pose, and consider how different the quality of your balance is in Child's Pose from the earlier poses. After a few minutes, sit on your mat, open your journal, and describe the different poses and how each influenced your feelings about balance.

▷ Standing on your mat, explore Tree Pose by lifting your foot to various heights, first only an inch or two, resting your heel against your standing leg while keeping your toes on the ground, then raising your foot a few inches, so the sole rests on your calf. Then move it to just below the knee, then to the inside of your upper thigh. Switch to the opposite foot and explore the pose again. Then come to Mountain Pose and feel the difference in balancing on two feet versus on one foot.

After a few breaths, sit down on your mat and use your journal to explore how you felt as you raised your foot higher and higher. How did the height influence your ability to find your balance? What changed? Were you able to find stillness even in the most challenging Tree Pose? Did you fall or lose your balance? Were you able to laugh about losing your balance and try again? Or were you upset because you weren't able to hold the pose? Write about your feelings in Tree Pose versus Mountain Pose. Which gave you more confidence? Which made you feel stronger? And which made you feel vulnerable? How did you find your balance after losing it?

➤ Sitting on your mat, open your journal and write about a situation in your life in which you lost your balance. Maybe it was a momentary flash of anger at a child for not following instructions or a brief moment of embarrassment over realizing that you'd forgotten to do something that you'd promised to do. What caused you to notice that your life was out of balance? And what steps did you take to regain your balance?

9: Learning to Breathe

Just recognizing your breath—knowing it's there—
is enough to help you find that calmness amidst the storm.
—FROM MY JOURNAL

At the core of our being and our practice is the breath. It's the way we begin each class, listening to our breath in the vocalization of *om*. And it's the way we end each class, listening again to the sound of our breath as we take in a deep inhalation and, releasing it, add our voice to the chorus of voices around of us. Each breath contains the key to our existence and the very mystery that is existence.

Within the span of ninety minutes, the length of our class, my breath changes, and changes again. In the beginning, it feels tight and unconnected to any rhythm. It's simply there, something that's part of my body even if I'm not aware of it. Taking in a deep breath and then releasing it slowly reminds me of its presence. The breath is there, part of life, just like the invisible force of energy that supports us in our poses, even when we're unable to see or feel it. For those first few minutes, I become conscious of my breath all over again, breathing in and out in a conscious rhythm, just to feel the breath fill my chest and lungs, just to hear it rasp and circle in the back of my throat as I breathe in and out.

Before we begin our series of poses, we sit quietly and set our foundations—twisting our thighs to increase the inner spiral, widening our sitting bones—and bring our hands to our hearts and take a deep breath and release it slowly, chanting *om*. The room suddenly comes alive with the sound of the breath connecting each of us with one another and with the source of energy out of which all life flows. How long you hold the *om* note is irrelevant. All that matters is that you feel your breath and sense the connection between your breath and the breath of everyone else in the room and the flow of energy emanating through it all.

FROM MY JOURNAL

The skin is only a temporary boundary, an illusion of separation. But, really, it's the connecting line between our inner and outer worlds. Maybe the distinction between inner and outer worlds is itself an illusion. Maybe there really is no distinction? Breathing is a dance that we're engaged in every moment of our lives: breathing in, breathing out.

I didn't always think of breathing that way. When I was younger and ran ten to fifteen miles a day, I took my breath for granted. It was something inside, almost disconnected from me, separate and apart. I knew that I needed to breathe in order to stay alive, but I didn't understand how my breath connected me to the world and to everyone in the world. I was too wrapped up in myself. All that mattered was running. And not just running, but running faster and longer than anyone else. There were times when I gasped for air, struggled for breath, wondered if I'd ever breathe easily again. After a strenuous race, I'd fall to my knees after crossing the finish line and feel as if my chest were going to explode if I didn't get enough air into my lungs. After a demanding practice, an afternoon training session, say, when we ran a series of steep hills to build our endurance, or repetitive quarter-mile laps around the track, I'd jog slowly, feeling my breath return to normal, leaving the zone that I'd managed to find while running, and I'd wonder if I would ever find my way into the zone again. I'd stand in the shower after returning to the locker room and breathe in the steam of the hot water and feel my chest expand and contract with my breath. But I didn't think about my breath as something that kept me alive, as something that connected me to the world. I wasn't even aware that such a connection between life and breath existed.

And yet I always loved seeing my breath puff out in front of me as I ran on cold mornings. I loved the feeling of being alive that running gave me, the tingling that I felt in my fingers and toes and on the surface of my skin as I ran, the intense joy that came from filling my lungs with air again and again and listening to the sound of air escaping and returning as I ran mile after mile. It was the breath that gave me the strength to run, but I didn't know it then.

Even now, long after I've stopped running, I can forget about my breath. During each pose, especially a challenging pose like Four-Limbed Staff Pose, I have to remind myself to breathe. It's natural in a challenging pose that pushes the limits of my strength to hold my breath without realizing it. But if I can remember to breathe, I can release some of that tension and explore the pose on an even deeper level, extending the limits or, at the very least, pushing against the boundary, so that one day I may be able to push a little further, go a little deeper.

FROM MY JOURNAL

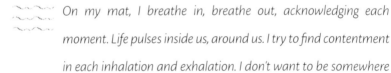 *On my mat, I breathe in, breathe out, acknowledging each moment. Life pulses inside us, around us. I try to find contentment in each inhalation and exhalation. I don't want to be somewhere else. Just here. Now.*

A bird calls outside the bedroom window. It's a bright red cardinal singing a series of sharp, long notes, then a quick succession of short whistles—maybe ten in all—before starting over again.

After mat: I didn't notice the time today. I didn't notice myself counting between breaths, just the breath itself. By the end of the session, I found my thoughts meandering rather than rushing. I could accept them, let them go, accept one more, let it go. Just watching. No judgment.

Each pose is different. Some test my limits, some open me up to new ways of viewing myself and feeling my breath, and some change over time, no longer as challenging as they once were. So Downward-Facing Dog Pose can feel more like a resting pose now than a difficult pose. And I notice how my breath, rather than being labored, comes more easily, in a regular rhythm, as I balance on all four limbs and stretch down my legs and up my spine and forearms.

But Warrior Pose II or Headstand quicken my breath—suddenly it sounds like a rushing waterfall—and I become conscious of just how essential it is to breathe, how crucial it is to my existence. As I come out of the challenging pose into Child's Pose I hear my breath differently, hear the gentle rhythm restored, feel it reviving my muscles, seeping into my bones, bringing rest.

Writing in my journal is like breathing onto the page. The words are physical evidence of my breath, my presence, mirrors of my inner spirit. After Rita handed out the journals to our class that morning long ago, I started making notes in it the moment that I reached my car, before driving away. One of my earliest entries describes breathing and how the breath can lead to the place where each of us needs to go to find our innermost selves. Ordinarily, I don't return to earlier entries, preferring to let them go, just like the breath, and move on. But as I was thinking about breathing and the process of keeping a journal, I returned to my old journal and found these:

FROM MY JOURNAL

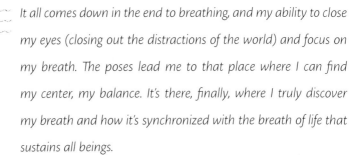

It all comes down in the end to breathing, and my ability to close my eyes (closing out the distractions of the world) and focus on my breath. The poses lead me to that place where I can find my center, my balance. It's there, finally, where I truly discover my breath and how it's synchronized with the breath of life that sustains all beings.

My limbs as they stretch and bend, my bones as they offer support, my muscles as they lift me above the earth and aid in my passage across the earth . . . through this life . . . and my senses and my mind—all are interconnected through the breath.

It's the breath, like the supply of blood, that keeps me alive, bringing oxygen into the system, letting my lungs expand and round and exhale. And it's the breath that accompanies the beating of my heart, the slow rhythm that pounds beneath my chest like a secret code, telling me that I'm alive.

It's the breath that lets me see the world. Not with my eyes, but with my inner eye, my intuition, my sense of how to live, which path to follow, whether I need to adjust a pose to attain my balance.

The breath reveals these secrets to me if I listen closely to it entering my body, bringing with it the wisdom of the ages, which has passed like the air itself from person to person, generation to generation, linking all those who have lived to all those who will live through the breath.

From My Journal

Think of the breath—inhaling and exhaling. Then, think of the way life seeps into the membranes of your cells and, then, leaks out again. If you listen to the rhythm of your breath, you can hear something else: the pulse of a life-force, larger than life itself, filling the universe with the same rhythm.

Then, think of the trees blowing in and bending out. Rain falling in slanted sheets, then drying in slick puddles. Sunlight disappearing behind a cloud, only to reappear in a blue sky. Think of the way life is always changing—even when you can't see it—between each breath. Before you can grasp it, the moment has fled, and another has replaced it, followed by another, and another.

The longer you listen to the rhythm of your breath, the more strongly compelled you are to view the line of separation between inner and outer as invisible.

It's such a powerful idea, the breath as unifying force, not only of your body but of your world beyond sight, beyond sense. Breathe gently, one breath after another. Listen to the sound of your breathing as you wake up and as you fall asleep, as you come into a pose and as you leave a pose. Notice the changes in your breath from moment to moment, hour to hour.

Listen: Your breath is telling you a secret. Open fully to each moment; embrace life as it flows through you. That moment of embrace is, I think, what we strive for when we step onto our yoga mat. And it's what we strive for when we step off the mat, too. We want to feel life fully, and, when we pass from this world to the next, following our breath, we want to be able to say: Yes, we have lived. Yoga lets me say this every time I practice. It reminds me that I am alive, that life offers such possibility of choices moment to moment, if only I choose to live them each fully.

It all begins with the breath. And it all ends with the breath. Between the end of an exhalation and beginning of the next inhalation, we pause in the space there and become the breath, the bridge between past and future, known and unknown, each breath leading us to a new pose, each pose helping us feel more and more alive in each moment.

Just like your breath, your journal will lead you where you need to go and will help you open up to the possibilities of life on and off the mat. And, like your breath, it will teach you what you need to know.

Journal Practice: Learning to Breathe

▶ Sit and breathe slowly, purposefully. Draw each breath deep into the back of your throat so that it fills your lungs, pause a moment or two, and then let it out deliberately. Listen to the sound your breath makes as you inhale and exhale. Listen to the rush of air, the steady stream, as it flows in and out. Feel your chest rise and fall. Notice how your stomach expands and contracts. Spend five minutes just sitting and breathing. What does breathing deeply, with intent, make you aware of? Does following your breath help you feel connected to a greater energy, a larger force? How do you feel when you pause between exhalation and inhalation, at the moment when you are breathing neither in nor out? Open your journal and describe what you notice.

▶ Notice that you can relax even in the most difficult of poses by focusing on your breath. It's true off the mat as well as on it. For instance, the next time you find yourself rushing to catch a plane or to get to your child's music recital, notice how your breath quickens; notice if you feel tenseness in your shoulders and your chest, if you feel cut off from yourself. When you find yourself straining in a challenging pose, notice how you have to remember to breathe, and notice that as soon as you become aware of your breath, your pose changes, your stomach relaxes, and your breath slows, even if you hold the pose a little longer. Take fifteen minutes to explore these issues in your journal. Write about a time when you felt rushed and out of control. And then write about a pose that you find challenging, almost impossible. What do these poses on and off the mat share in common? How are they different? Imagine yourself in a challenging situation and notice your breath. Then, as you stay in that challenging place, remember to breathe deeply. How does breathing deeply alter your relationship to the situation?

▸ Go for a walk in the woods or in a city park; stroll on the beach or down a quiet street. Listen to the sound of the wind, the steady rush of the waves, or the leaves of a nearby tree, and try to breathe in rhythm to the sounds of nature. Then find a quiet place to reflect on the quality of wind or air or waves and how the breath contains and reflects similar elements. Describe what you feel as you breathe in rhythm with the wind or the waves. Can you feel a larger energy or force linking you to the natural world? Can you feel that same energy or force inside yourself?

▸ Listen to your breath. Just breathe deeply and listen. If you're alone, imagine that you're in a room full of people breathing beside you. If you're in a room full of people, imagine that you're alone. How does your breath change when you're alone? How does it change when you're with people? Write about what you hear in each situation. Try not to judge one as better or worse, just examine the quality of your breath, the depth of each inhalation, the sounds that take you deeper into the breath and the sounds that distract you, the challenge of taking longer breaths, the pivoting space when you pause between breaths. What do you notice? Can you breathe into different parts of your body? Again, ask yourself what you notice. When you're done writing, put down your pen and close your journal. Just breathe for a minute or two. Let your breath flow in its natural rhythm, and let that rhythm carry over into your life.

10: Listening to Your Voice

No judgment, no praise, no criticism—
just words on a page—that let me see myself in a new light.
—FROM MY JOURNAL

At the end of our session in December 2007, after studying with
Rita for more than a year, I learned that she was leaving the
studio to care for her aging parents. So, with some trepidation, I
signed up for the class that Jaye was offering on Monday mornings at 10. I was sorry to be leaving Rita's Tuesday morning class,
a place where I'd learned to listen to and trust my voice. Would
I still be able to hear my voice? Would I still be able to trust it?
Or would Jaye's voice overpower and drown it out?

Stepping into Jaye's class on that Monday morning in January,
I felt like I was a beginning student again. I had no idea where
the next twelve weeks would lead me, no idea what poses or
themes Jaye was planning to teach, no idea if I had the strength
or skill or fundamental understanding of my own body to be
able to do the poses. I walked into the class fearful of what I

might find out about myself, about my ability to pursue questions and meet challenges, worried about meeting new people, my shyness, as always, a constant companion. As I entered the class, I realized that I was hearing my old voice again, the voice of doubt and anxiety and cowardice, and I had to laugh. I hadn't heard that voice for so long, I'd almost forgotten that it was part of me. Over the sessions with Rita, I'd learned how to find a new voice, a voice that came from a different source within me, a voice filled with confidence and courage.

It had taken years to uncover that voice, to understand that my voice was made up of many layers, and that the layers were fed by many emotions, the way underground streams feed into a larger river. Rita had helped draw this voice out of me by handing me a journal. If I doubted its existence, all I had to do was to open my journal and read a passage or two that I'd written a day or a week or a year ago. So, as I stepped onto the mat to begin Jaye's class that morning, I imagined myself opening the pages of my journal and leafing through them to read some of the passages, and I could hear the new voice coming through the pages. It provided the support that I needed at that moment.

I quieted my anxieties by paying attention to my breath flowing in and out. I focused on what I love most about being at the yoga center—the sense of freedom that I don't find anywhere else except in the poses. I found that by paying attention to my breath I could stop worrying about my performance and how other people might judge me. I could view each pose that we would try as a new exploration of the world, a process of uncovering things about myself and my relationships with people that I might not have known before.

Jaye gathered us in a circle on that first morning and began by asking us to commit to what we love. "You'll find stability in your life," he said, "because loving what you do will bring less resistance and more desire."

Commit to what you love. The words echoed in my head and heart, and I had to smile. That is what I'd done by registering for this class. Hearing him say these words quieted my doubts and made me feel that I'd made the right choice, that my voice of faith and hope and courage had led me here to Jaye's class for a reason that I had yet to discover. I closed my eyes and breathed with greater ease as I listened to Jaye and waited for the asana practice to begin.

As Jaye led us through our opening series of poses, I focused my attention on what I love—my wife, my daughter, my father, my brother, my work—and was surprised to find how much my stability increased in each pose and how much stronger and confident my voice became. No longer did I hear the doubts and fears, only the steady sound of my breath in and out as I flowed from pose to pose, and a voice from deep in my heart whispering: Commit to what you love. Why should that be, I wondered? How does love, just thinking about love, increase our strength and stability? And why does focusing on what we love allow us to gain confidence as the pose becomes more challenging the longer we hold it? In each new pose, I felt my heart beating and could feel the blood flowing through my limbs, and I knew that the students on either side of my mat could feel the same thing. Somehow, in some mysterious way, the love that I felt was supporting them in their poses, just as the love that they felt was supporting me in mine. We were linked by the invisible threads of our lives and by our breath. And even though we were strangers to each other in that first class, I felt as if we knew each other through the pulse of our hearts, the inhalation and exhalation of our breath. We shared the same space, the same air, the same earth, and our voices all sang silently a hymn to what we loved.

FROM MY JOURNAL

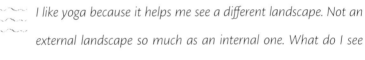 *I like yoga because it helps me see a different landscape. Not an external landscape so much as an internal one. What do I see today?*

A rose that my wife gave me last week. Every day the flower changes, becomes more beautiful than the day before. No, not more beautiful; just beautiful in a different way than the day before, in a way that I hadn't expected.

It's the same with our lives, isn't it? Days unfold like petals, blossoming, reaching toward a source we cannot see. And we draw nutrients up through our roots, see beauty through our eyes, hear it with our ears, taste it with our lips, and touch it with our fingertips.

It's the same with our relationship, which grows lovelier as we grow older. There is beauty, just as there are thorns. Joy and pain. Each is contained in the life that we share together.

With the rose you can see the daily changes: how the petals curl and shift color; how the flower opens and widens; how it begins to droop a little on the neck of the stem. Life's changes aren't as obvious. But they're there all the same. They take place even when we're unaware of them. The rose reminds me to look closer. Pay attention, I tell myself. I don't want to miss a thing.

Most of the poses that Jaye introduced in our class over the next twelve weeks were versions of the poses that I'd become familiar with in Rita's class, but he asked us to hold the poses longer. Each time that I thought I'd reached my limit, I heard a voice coming from my well of doubts saying that I'd done enough, was straining too hard, had reached the end of my strength, and should give up. And I'd have to reach down a little deeper for an ounce more of strength and push past that voice of protest until I heard another voice rising from my heart, as the sweat poured off my arms and legs—a voice of encouragement, of support, a voice whispering that I had the strength to go further, possessed the stamina to hold the pose for another breath, could summon the courage to go to a place I'd never been before. I would close my eyes and breathe deeply and try to remain open to the possibility of holding the pose another second, and then another, and another, and I could feel myself stretching and expanding into the unknown.

Some of the poses required greater dexterity and balance than I had yet mastered, and I struggled to stay on my feet, strained to hear my voice and find the confidence to listen to it without losing my balance and crashing to the floor. Some of the students on mats nearest mine made the poses look effortless, while others struggled like me to find a way to ease into the pose. And I realized, as I struggled in the poses, that my critical voice was constantly comparing my ability and performance to others, always competing, wanting to be the best or the strongest or the fastest. I listened to that voice and acknowledged it, accepting without judgment the part of me that felt that way, and then, as before, I let go of those feelings, and turned inward. I listened for a voice that rose out of a different place, a voice that encouraged me to explore the pose without fear of embarrassment, a voice that told me it wasn't a performance. No one was judging how I stood on the mat. No one cared whether I held my balance or not. Holding my balance, the voice assured me, was irrelevant. What was relevant was exploring the idea of balance. Find a way to keep your balance in the face of challenges, whispered the voice. Each time we entered into another challenging pose, I listened to that voice.

As we explored different poses in class together, I realized that Jaye was no longer the obstacle that I'd feared but rather a helpful guide whose insights into yoga and life gave me a new way of understanding myself and my voice. Each time we entered an unfamiliar pose, I found myself comforted rather than intimidated by his presence. I welcomed the moments in class when he pointed out areas where I needed to adjust my stance in, say, Mountain Pose, or when I might benefit from clawing my fingertips more firmly into the mat in Downward-Facing Dog Pose or puffing out the space around my kidneys while upside down in Headstand. Jaye described each asana and then demonstrated it before we attempted it ourselves. I could see each pose in my mind before I stepped into it because his instructions were so precise. Instead of drowning out my voice, his words helped clarify my understanding of the pose. By encouraging me to take risks, to explore new territory in each pose, he helped me hear my own voice more clearly. "Try it," he'd say whenever he noticed my hesitation. "You have nowhere you need to go, nothing else you need to do. Just have fun with it."

In his class, as in Rita's, I learned that yoga could be fun, a way of seeing the world and myself that was limitless. I found myself less worried about what would happen from week to week. The critical, judgmental voice seemed to accept, finally, that I'd found another way of looking at the world, another voice to listen to, and it fell silent, although at times I could still hear it complaining that I wasn't giving it the proper attention or time to voice its protests fully. I'd listen to it for a few moments, but the voice had grown weaker and less insistent. It was no longer the force that it had once been. When I listened for it, I heard a whimper rather than a shout.

It was in Jaye's class that I began to see how each of us chooses the voice that we hear, the voice that we want to listen to. It's not quite as easy as tuning a radio to the AM or FM station that you'd like to hear. But it is like tuning in to a voice that helps you understand the world and yourself rather than a voice that clouds your world (and yourself) with doubt, fear, and anxiety. Our ability to choose is one of the lessons that Jaye imparts to his students. Each of us, he says, has a choice to make in how we practice yoga. Just as we choose how we keep our journals or how we live our lives, we can choose, too, to conceal our true voices or reveal them. The choice is in our power. We only have to find the courage to make it.

What I've found in the process of keeping a journal and practicing yoga is that to hear your voice, it's essential that you go beyond yourself, reach beyond the limits that you might have set (unknowingly) for yourself. It's where I heard my voice for the first time: in that pause between thinking I'd gone far enough, held a pose long enough, and compelling myself to take another breath and hold the pose a second or two longer.

Some weeks it takes a day or two for my muscles to recover from such strenuous exertions. A skilled yogi is able to recognize the difference between stiffness and discomfort (which may come from exploring the edges of her limits) and pain (which is likely a sign that she may have exceeded her limits). Slightly sore or stiff muscles are signs of growth, I think, and increasing strength. Pain—sharp or dull, short-lived or long-lasting—is a sign of overworking, pushing too hard. Greater strength will help me the next time I step on the mat to hold Lunge Pose or Four-Limbed Staff Pose with more awareness, kick into Headstand with less effort, and learn how to be myself with greater ease. In each instance, when I face a new challenge and push toward my limits, I have to trust the voice that I discovered in the pages of my journal. It can guide me away from fear and doubt toward greater energy and strength.

That trust only comes with time. It's part of the mystery of practicing yoga and writing. In each class, on each page, I learn another way to be myself, to hear my voice, to reach unafraid into the unknown. Each pose builds on the poses that I learned in previous classes, expanding my understanding of how the practice of yoga can bring me more fully into each moment. Each page helps me become a fuller expression of who I am now.

Lately Jaye talks a lot about trusting our voices, our inner teachers. "Listen to your breath. It's what links you to your inner teacher." His words echo in my mind long after I leave his class. *Inner teacher. Inner teacher.* Is this what my yoga practice over the past few years and writing in my journal day after day have helped me do? Have they taught me how to listen to my inner teacher?

FROM MY JOURNAL

The writing lets me touch something inside me—reach a place only accessible when a pen and journal are at hand. It's there, inside me, all the time, but the key to opening the door and stepping inside is the pen and paper. Without seeing the words on paper, without the physical act of writing, there's something vaguely abstract and elusive about one's thoughts whereas w/ pen and paper we make those thoughts concrete—bring them into the light—and that process of finding out what you think is not just liberating, it's self-affirming—and gives you a way to know yourself on a deeper, more intimate level—because in the writing process you discover things you didn't even realize you

knew or were thinking. They just appear—as if by magic—as if
somehow your inner guide, your own inner wisdom—was given
permission to speak—and you listened and heard and were
present to write it down—and you can choose to read it later or
not, or to just bask in the glow of the inner light that shines out
when you sit on the mat and take pen and paper in your lap

Journal Practice: Listening to Your Voice

▶ One of the greatest challenges of listening to your own voice is noticing the differences between your critical voice and your nurturing voice. In the former, you'll hear expectations of what should be, and in the latter you'll hear what your voice sounds like without any expectations.

To notice the difference between these two voices, sit on your mat with your journal, and write down two questions on two different pages. On the first page, write: "Who do others expect me to be?" And on the second page: "Who am I?" Both questions will help you begin to understand the difference between the voice that you create in response to expectations and the voice that comes without expectations from the deepest part of yourself, your natural voice.

If you have trouble sitting with these questions, begin your asana practice, and notice in each pose the voices that you hear as you flow from one pose to the next. Does the voice seem to come from outside yourself? Does it set expectations in the pose that you feel you need to meet? And simultaneously do you notice another, softer voice, a voice that encourages you to explore the pose? Notice how you feel moment to moment as each pose unfolds. After you finish your asana practice, take your journal and pen and describe how these two voices sound. What does it feel like when you hear each voice?

Describe the voices that you heard in the various poses— the voice of expectation, of acceptance, of denial or disagreement or shame, of contentment, and the voice of pure joy. Focus on the voice of expectation for a moment. Can you identify the source of the voice? Can you define the expectations? How does this voice make you feel? And how does it differ from the voice of acceptance, say, or the voice of contentment?

Now write about the challenges of hearing your natural voice. Why is it harder to hear on some days and easier on other days? Describe how it feels to sit with your natural voice.

▶ Your voice can serve as a catalyst for change, but only if you're willing to welcome change rather than resist it. By noticing how you feel about change, you may gain insights into your voice and your approach to life.

Sit for a few moments with your journal in your lap, and consider how you feel about changes in your life. Do you welcome change? Resist it? Do you seek ways to avoid change? Now, think of an example that reflects how you respond to change. As you tell yourself—or imagine telling someone else—about the example, do you hear tension or relief in your voice? Describe how your voice sounds in a situation when change is inevitable—a change in job, a child's graduation from high school, a death in the family. Write about how the change made you feel. Did you welcome or resist the change?

Can you see a link between your reluctance to try a backbend, for instance, and your inability or unwillingness to welcome change? If you're tight in your shoulders, are you willing to explore ways to open yourself up? Or do you prefer to stay tight and try to ignore the tightness? Is the tightness reflected in your voice? Imagine how your voice might sound in an open space, and then write about the different way your voice sounds in an open rather than a constricted space.

A week or so later, reread your entry. Take a few minutes to write about how you feel now about change. Note if your feelings are different and if your voice is different since the last time you reflected on change. If it's too painful to reread your earlier entry, reflect in your journal about your feelings toward rereading your work.

11: Becoming Your Own Teacher

I keep telling myself: It's not a question of "can't"
but rather "not yet."
—FROM MY JOURNAL

You never know where life will lead you or who you'll find to help you on your way. Somehow, though, as we make our way through life, we find the teachers who help us in our practice and in life, just when we need them most. They appear in our lives as if by magic and support us as we grope in the dark to find our path. Over the course of my life, each of my teachers has illuminated a little more of the path stretching ahead of me, helping me see just enough to go a little further. Now, after more than five years of practicing yoga, I enter into poses that once struck me as nearly impossible, poses that I never thought I'd be able to do on my own—Headstand, Handstand, Forearm Balance. I can kick up into Handstand or step into Headstand without needing a wall for support. And though I can't remain inverted for long, I can find a way to relax in the pose. Upside down, feeling the blood rush to my head, I puff out my lower back, stretch my feet to the sky, and extend my spine upward through the soles of my feet and downward into my skull while breathing deeply.

In one sense, the distance that I've traveled over the past five years to learn how to do such poses isn't far. Our class meets in the same cinder-block building overlooking the same pond. The same mats and blocks are stored in the same closets; the same blankets are folded and stacked on the same shelves; the same belts dangle from the same hooks. And it takes the same amount of time to drive to the yoga center (except if a flock of migrating sandhill cranes happens to be blocking the road).

But, in another sense, the distance is enormous. The world may appear the same, but my perspective, my ability to look at and see the world, has changed. Over the past few years, the practice of keeping a journal has sharpened my senses, helped me learn to trust my intuition, and made me more attuned to the process of life and the way an unseen, invisible force guides the universe. I have faith that that force, that energy, will support me in my life, just as it supports me in my yoga practice, a faith that I didn't have or wasn't aware of before I began keeping a practice journal.

FROM MY JOURNAL

Following the breath requires that thoughts and motion slow down. You have to assume a pattern natural to your own body.

In this way the breath becomes your teacher. Listen to your breath, and you can begin to understand your body: what your body needs; how close or far you are from the source at the core of your being; whether or not you are in balance.

Yoga is striving for balance, an exploration of what balance is, and an attempt to achieve balance in your life. You can't rush growth anymore than you can rush the natural rhythm of your breath. Growth and understanding come when they come, not before.

Each of my yoga teachers has helped open my eyes to a different stage of the process. In their own way, as they encouraged me to explore new poses, they helped me discover new and different sides of myself. Vesna taught me patience and how to let go of fear. Her gentle voice prompted me to relax and ease into each pose, to root myself in the moment, to close my eyes and listen to my breath.

Jaye taught me how to look more closely at each pose, to find the focal points (the upper palate, the heart, or the pelvis) that would bear the weight of each asana so I could understand the structure of the pose. In the process of exploring each pose and its focal point, he helped me recognize the difference between my physical heart and my spiritual heart. Thanks to him, I'm learning how to strengthen my foundation, the values and principles on which I try to build my life, not just on the mat but off the mat as well.

Rita helped me rediscover the joy that I thought I'd lost years ago. Her willingness to experiment and lead us in playful poses helped me regain a sense of the possibilities that life offers, and her constant good cheer in the face of her own personal difficulties restored my faith in life, as well as my trust that life would bring me what I needed when I most needed it.

Once I might have thought it was an accident that I found Rita and Jaye and the yoga center when I needed to learn lessons about courage and integrity and teamwork and love of life and writing. Now I'm not so sure. The universe is listening, I think. It gives you what you really need if you know how to listen.

FROM MY JOURNAL

 Yoga—the practice of poses, learning how to come into a pose and how to accept where I am in the pose—has proven an effective teacher in my writing practice. Just knowing where you are is a remarkable discovery, never mind understanding where you've been or where you're going. You can't live in the past, and you can't see the future. You can only set your place mindfully in the present and project your thoughts toward a place where you might want to see yourself in a day or a week, then pull back to the present and work toward that goal, as if it's a distant mountain that you might reach one day.

There's a kind of beauty in patience. Can you accept the

pace of your life as it unfolds in its own shape and at its own deliberate timetable? Life is not in our control as much as within our control. We can influence and shape life, but a larger force is the driving element behind our actions. It's that force, that energy, which each pose brings us in closer touch with.

What's the next stage in my journey? I don't know. Perhaps, if I listen closely enough, I'll find the answer on my mat or in the pages of my journal. In class each Monday morning, Jaye keeps inspiring me to reach for and try to understand new aspects of myself. His passion and enthusiasm for yoga and life remind me that joy can be found in the process of trying rather than in the actual arriving. "That's because you'll always arrive at some other place," Jaye says, "another pose you haven't yet mastered, another obstacle, another unexpected challenge." I'm coming to understand and accept this process as the never-ending asana of life. And in the process I'm becoming my own teacher.

Afterword:
Wherever the Path Leads

....

As I write these words, I can barely move the tip of my tongue to touch the molars on the lower right side of my mouth. During conversations, especially over the phone, if I slur a word or if my voice sounds hoarse or fades away altogether, I have to remind myself not to feel embarrassed. And when I take a sip of water or bite into a tuna salad sandwich, I have to remember that I may choke if I take too large a swallow or too big a bite.

The way I talk and swallow now—with the right side of my tongue, throat muscles, and vocal chords partially paralyzed—is different than the way I swallowed and talked four months ago. After weeks of tests—two MRIs, a lumbar puncture, a cerebral angiogram, and a CT scan—doctors discovered a tumor at the base of my skull which wasn't there when I finished an earlier draft of this book.

It took a base skull specialist and a neuroradiologist at the University of Florida's Shands Hospital in Gainesville to diagnose the problem correctly. The doctor explained that the

....

tumor was a benign Schwannoma arising out of the sheath of Schwann cells encasing the nerve. Its mass was pressing on my twelfth cranial nerve (and possibly on the ninth and tenth cranial nerves, as well), which was the reason why my tongue, throat muscles, and vocal chords no longer functioned the way they used to.

The tests were daunting, especially the cerebral angiogram, where I had to lie awake while a doctor inserted a catheter into my femoral artery and, once inside the aortic arch above my heart, injected dye into the arteries leading into the brain. Each was a test of forbearance and inner strength, as well as patience, and taking those tests was a journey that I never expected to make. But, amazingly, the experience turned into a journey of love and friendship rather than one of pain and fear, thanks to the care and kindness of strangers, family, and friends, and because keeping a journal and practicing yoga had taught me how to keep my perspective balanced.

I could have viewed the tumor and its effects as a crisis or as a sign of imminent mortality. Instead, I focused on my breath and could look at each day, each encounter (with doctors, nurses, lab technicians, radiologists, and even the hospital volunteers who wheeled me to exits after my procedures) as a gift, each moment a chance to make a new connection with another person helping me in my pose as patient (and human being).

On the days when I wasn't visiting doctors or taking tests, I stepped onto the mat to do my yoga practice, but that presented another kind of challenge. My muscles were so weak (the weakness, not quite gone, is still a mystery), I could barely hold Downward-Facing Dog Pose or Plank Pose for more than a few seconds, and I could no longer do inversions without feeling the back of my head start to throb. But easy stretches and twists, as well as lying quietly, eyes closed, in Relaxation Pose, helped me see the world anew and see myself—even with my new disability—as a work in progress, always changing, never the same.

Four months ago, when I first had trouble swallowing, I never imagined one day that my idea of perfection might be living with a partially paralyzed tongue, throat, and vocal chords. That was before I learned that I had a tumor, before my wife insisted on accompanying me to each procedure, each test, each doctor's appointment, before the two of us celebrated our twentieth anniversary in the hospital on the day that I underwent a lumbar puncture. That procedure, as well as all the other tests (and waiting for the results), gave us a chance to appreciate our love for each other. And our yoga practice helped us let go of the past, release our worries about a future we might not have, and appreciate the moments that we shared. In these shared moments we found a kind of perfection.

I have the strength now to go on a two-mile walk each morning, to take deep breaths of fresh air and feel my heart beating and admire the sun rising above the trees. I may have impaired speech and a hoarse voice and difficulty swallowing, but I still feel gratitude for the blueness of the sky, the touch of the wind on my skin, the taste of salt air on my lips. I am still me. And as I unroll my mat in class again—a gentle restorative class with Vesna, my first yoga teacher—and begin to do my series of poses, I can feel myself surrounded by people who love me for who I am, regardless of the form my body may take in this moment or the shape-shifting it may undergo in the future. Each of us will age, and each of us will change in some unpredictable and unforeseen way as the years pass. All of us are changing right now, even if we're unaware of it.

Sometimes it takes a lifetime to find perfection. But keeping a journal and practicing yoga have helped me find perfection in the kindness and love that we bestow on each other every day. I found it in my wife's love, and in the devotion of a brother who flew down one weekend to join us amidst the onslaught of tests, and in the prayers of distant friends whose phone calls and letters provided unexpected support throughout the months of uncertainty. I found it in the unexpected kindnesses of strangers, as well as in the care and concern of teachers like Rita and Jaye, and in the unstinting generosity of friends like Paula, one of the students in my class with Rita long ago, who is now my wife's teacher.

One day, as I was concluding this chapter, Paula surprised me by sending home a gift with my wife. Inside a bright orange plastic bag that my wife set down on the kitchen table were three blank journals. The journals, each a different size, were wrapped in a wide, emerald-green ribbon, and, tucked with care under a large green bow, was a note in Paula's neat handwriting urging me to keep writing.

Along with the journals and the note, Paula sent a small white cardboard box, the kind that usually contains earrings or some sort of jewelry. When I lifted the lid, I found inside an ordinary bottle cap. On the bottom of the cap were these words:

"The pen is mightier than the sword and considerably easier to write with."
—Marty Feldman

And I laughed a hearty laugh because Paula had helped me see the situation—and my new challenges—with a sense of humor.

Holding the journals in my hands that afternoon, I was reminded of how much I love writing and journals and the blank pages waiting for a pen to fill the empty space with words. I wondered what I might say, wondered who I might share the words with, wondered about the path my life might take and where the journals might lead me. After four months of illness, the world was filling with possibility again.

Friends have suggested that I should write about my experiences over the past four months. Maybe I will one day, but not yet; it's still a little soon for me. I prefer getting into the water and swimming around a while, getting a sense of balance, a sense of where I am, before swimming in any one direction. It took five years, after all, to begin writing about yoga and for this book to emerge from the jottings and scribbling in my journals.

Now, as I come to the end of this book, I have no idea what the next moment will bring. But I do know that these new journals, these gifts from Paula, will help me find my way. They offer hope and remind me that I can write for as long as my mind and body allow me to keep practicing—in my journal and on my mat.

Resources

This list of resources is hardly comprehensive; it's simply a collection of material that I came across by chance as I followed the path that led me here. Now, looking back over my shoulder at my trail, I can see that my tracks form a zigzag pattern or, more accurately, a series of concentric circles expanding outward. Rarely, if ever, did I take a straight line. But straight lines—their speed, their efficiency—are overrated. It's the meandering paths, the ones that take us into the unknown and back again, that give us the opportunity to make discoveries. By the time I finished this book, I no longer cared if my path was straight or zigzagged. What mattered wasn't the goal, after all, but the journey that brought me here. I hope this collection of resources proves helpful to you, as well. Write and let me know when you get a chance.

Namaste,
Bruce Black
bruceblack@ymail.com

A few websites and books on keeping a journal that may help you get started:

Journal Writing
www.journal-writing.com
An online workshop that will take you step-by-step through the process of writing a journal.

Writing the Journey
www.writingthejourney.com
A collection of resources on keeping journals, including journal writing exercises, feature articles, and book recommendations.

The 1000 Journals Project
www.1000journals.com
An online experiment in collaborative journal writing.

Journal for You
www.journalforyou.com
A treasure trove of articles and advice on keeping a journal.

Journaling Life
www.journalinglife.com
Over thirty different journal styles—from gardening and diet to prayer and gratitude—with samples and suggestions for ideas on how to choose a journal style suitable for you.

Writing Yoga with Bruce Black

http://journalpractice.wordpress.com

Join me on my blog, where I share excerpts from my journal and offer writing exercises to help you keep one of your own.

Wordswimmer

http://wordswimmer.blogspot.com

In my blog on the writing process, named one of the Web's "Top 100 Creative Writing Blogs" and included in "100 Great Blogs That Young Writers Should Read," you'll find essays on the craft of writing, as well as interviews with writers on the writing process.

Teachers are an invaluable part of the writing process. You can study with some of the finest by going into your local bookstore or library and checking out their work. Here are a few who I admire :

Natalie Goldberg

www.nataliegoldberg.com

Goldberg's *Writing Down the Bones* has become a classic text for helping writers understand the writing process. She offers numerous books, workshops, and tapes to nurture writers seeking a deeper understanding of the process.

Julia Cameron

www.theartistsway.com

Cameron's *The Artist's Way*, like Goldberg's work, encourages writers to reach their full potential as creative artists. Her books have inspired many writers, and her website offers some basic tools for you to begin your journey.

Gail Sher

www.gailsher.com

Sher, an accomplished poet, writer, teacher, and psychotherapist, practices Tibetan Buddhism and offers unique insights into writing as a practice.

Nothing can replace choosing a journal by picking it up and feeling its weight in your hand, opening it, and touching its pages. But if you can't find what you want at your local stationary store or bookstore, you may want to go online to find a journal. Here are some sources:

Etsy

www.etsy.com/category/paper_goods/journal

A site where you can find a variety of handmade journals.

Journaling Arts

www.journalingarts.com

An online resource for journal lovers.

Jenni Bick Bookbinding
www.jennibick.com
A collection of custom-designed journals.

Nomad Journals
www.nomadjournals.com
Journals designed especially for outdoor activities.

These yoga teachers and their books helped me think more deeply about yoga and the interconnectedness of yoga and life. They inspired me in my practice, and I hope they'll inspire you, too:

Judith Hanson Lasater
www.judithlasater.com
My wife took a yoga workshop with Judith Hanson Lasater and purchased her book, *Living Your Yoga*, which she shared with me. It was Judith's book that helped me glimpse how what I was learning on the mat might apply to the events of my daily life.

Donna Farhi
www.donnafarhi.co.nz
Donna Farhi is one of America's most respected yoga teachers, and her book *Bringing Yoga to Life* is, like Lasater's, a life-transforming guide to how yoga can serve as a foundation for navigating the challenges of life.

Stephen Cope

www.kripalu.org/article/581

Cope is the author of *The Wisdom of Yoga*, a book that helped explain some of the history, background, and mystery of yoga as I struggled to learn some of its poses. He teaches at Kripalu, a retreat center where you can find a variety of yoga practices suitable for your skill level.

Erich Schiffmann

www.movingintostillness.com

Schiffmann is the author of *Moving into Stillness*, and his website gives readers the chance to explore his book.

Rita Knorr

www.fulcrumblu.com

This is Rita's website, where you can meet the teacher who gave me the journal that led to *Writing Yoga*. You'll find a wealth of information about yoga in the lessons she's posted to help students develop a home practice.

John Friend

www.anusara.com

Everything you want to know about Anusara Yoga and John Friend, its founder, can be found on this website, including a helpful directory of teachers who practice Anusara Yoga in your neighborhood.

Betsey Downing

www.gardenoftheheartyoga.com

This is the Garden of the Heart Yoga Center website, where you can read more about Betsey and Jaye and some of the teachers who helped shape my yoga practice. If you're ever in Sarasota, why not drop in for a sample class?

A small sampling of the yoga resources that you'll find online:

Body and Breath

www.bodyandbreath.com

A site that explores the anatomy and physiology of hatha yoga, including discussions of breathing exercises, abdominal exercises, pelvic exercises, standing postures, backward bending postures, forward bending postures, twisting postures, Headstand, Shoulderstand, and meditation.

Hugger Mugger

www.huggermugger.com

You'll find a remarkable array of yoga accessories—from blocks, belts and mats to DVDs, jewelry, and designer yoga clothes—at this well-known site to help you feel (and look) good in your practice

The Secrets of Yoga

www.thesecretsofyoga.com

A comprehensive resource of articles, equipment, teacher directory, retreats, and more.

Yoga Basics

www.yogabasics.com

A helpful resource for learning the basic poses, along with information on the history and philosophy of different types of yoga.

YogaDork

www.yogadork.com

My editor brought this site to my attention, and although I'm not a committed YogaDork, I can see why she loves checking this hipster-ish blog, with its edgy sense of humor and up-to-the-minute commentary on what's happening in today's yoga community.

Yoga Journal

www.yogajournal.com

The online edition of the popular magazine offers videos, articles, tips on practice, etc.

Yoga Network

www.yoganetwork.co.uk

Another resource to answer basic questions about yoga poses and the different types of yoga practiced today.

About the Author

Bruce Black began studying yoga five years ago, when his knees could no longer stand the stress of running. After taking classes for a few years, he began keeping a journal to explore his experiences on the mat. Out of his journal and his devotion to Anusara Yoga emerged *Writing Yoga*, a book that explores the nexus of yoga, writing, and life.

A graduate of Columbia University, where he received a BA in English literature, he earned his MFA in writing from Vermont College (now Vermont College of Fine Arts). His stories have appeared in *Cricket* and *Cobblestone* magazines and other publications, and his blog, *Wordswimmer*, was named one of the Web's "Top 100 Creative Writing Blogs" by Online Education News and is included in Online Degrees Hub's list of "100 Great Blogs That Young Writers Should Read."

He serves as a poetry judge for The Cybils: Children's and Young Adult Bloggers' Literacy Awards and is the founder and editorial director of The Jewish Writing Project.

He lives with his wife and daughter in Sarasota, Florida, where he teaches writing workshops for children and adults and spends most of his time, when he's not reading or writing in his journal, practicing Tree Pose. You can visit him at *Wordswimmer,* his blog on writing (http://wordswimmer.blogspot.com) or *Writing Yoga with Bruce Black,* his blog on keeping a journal (http://journalpractice.wordpress.com), or write to him at bruceblack@ymail.com.

From the Publisher

Shambhala Publications is pleased to publish the Rodmell Press collection of books on yoga, Buddhism, and aikido. As was the aspiration of the founders of Rodmell Press, it is our hope that these books will help individuals develop a more skillful practice—one that brings peace to their daily lives and to the Earth.

To learn more, please visit www.shambhala.com.

Printed in the United States
by Baker & Taylor Publisher Services